The
Super
ANTIOXIDANT
DIET
and Nutrition Guide

The Super ANTIOXIDANT DIET and Nutrition Guide

A Health Plan for the Body, Mind, and Spirit

ROBIN JEEP AND RICHARD COUEY, PHD,
with Sherie Pitman Ellington

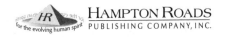
HAMPTON ROADS
PUBLISHING COMPANY, INC.
for the evolving human spirit

The Super Antioxidant Diet and Nutrition Guide
A Health Plan for Body, Mind, and Spirit

Robin Jeep and Richard Bryant Couey, PhD, with Sherie Pitman Ellington

Cover design by Frame25 Productions
Cover art by David G. Freund Photography, c/o Istock;
Rafal Zdeb, c/o Istock; Marlee90, c/o Istock;
Andrew F. Kazmierski, c/o Shutterstock; Liv friis-larsen, c/o Shutterstock

Hampton Roads Publishing Company, Inc.
1125 Stoney Ridge Road
Charlottesville, VA 22902

434-296-2772 • fax: 434-296-5096
e-mail: hrpc@hrpub.com • www.hrpub.com

If you are unable to order this book from your local
bookseller, you may order directly from the publisher.
Call 1-800-766-8009, toll-free.

Library of Congress Cataloging-in-Publication Data

Jeep, Robin, 1954-
  The super antioxidant diet and nutrition guide : a health plan for body,
mind, and spirit / Robin Jeep and Richard Bryant Couey ; with Sherie Pitman
Ellington.
      p. cm.
  Includes bibliographical references and index.
  Summary: "Advocates a diet rich in vegetables, with limited meat intake.
Includes exercise plan and more than 70 healthful recipes"--Provided by
publisher.
  ISBN-13: 978-1-57174-557-6 (7 x 9 tp : alk. paper)
  1. Nutrition. 2. Antioxidants. I. Couey, Richard B. II. Ellington,
Sherie Pitman. III. Title.
  RA784.J44 2008
  613.2--dc22

                    2007043157

ISBN 978-1-57174-557-6
10 9 8 7 6 5 4 3 2 1
Printed on acid-free paper in Canada

NOTE TO THE READER

The Super Antioxidant Diet has been designed for the average person who loves good food and wants to achieve optimal health. The diet is powerful, and following it will change your life. As with any lifestyle change, however, you are encouraged to consult your physician first. If you have any type of medical condition[*] or illness, you should be supervised by a medical doctor with a background in nutrition. No dietary plan can guarantee a complete reversal of disease or serve as a substitute for professional medical care.

[*]*Caution: Insulin diabetics may experience a severe drop in their blood glucose while on this diet. Diabetics should be under the supervision of their physician and closely monitor their glucose levels while following this diet plan.*
—Richard B. Couey, PhD

I dedicate this book to my Father, the Father of lights, the Giver of gifts, and the Lover of my soul; to my parents, who gave me natural life; to Bobby, my twin, who shared part of that life; to Philip, who nurtured me back to life; to my daughter, Alexandra, who brought me the joy of life; to Y'shua (Jesus), who gave me true life, which is the light of the world.

CONTENTS

FOREWORD

There is no subject of greater physiological importance or more vital to the welfare of the human race than the subject of nutrition. How best to maintain the body in a condition of health and strength, and how to establish the highest degree of efficiency physically, spiritually, and mentally are questions of nutrition that every enlightened person should explore. We hear widely divergent views from nearly everyone regarding the needs of the body and the extent of our daily nutritional requirements. We find contradictory statements as to the relative merit of animal and vegetable foods. There is a lack of agreement regarding many of the fundamental issues that arise in any consideration of the nutrition needs of the human body. This is especially true regarding the food requirements of a healthy adult.

Robin Jeep has immersed herself in the study of the latest scientific evidence regarding nutrition, exercise, and stress and its impact on the chemistry of the human cell. In this book, she presents a clear and practical understanding of how health can be achieved by obtaining homeostasis in the cell. She shows that most diseases are caused by poor nutrition and she reveals how eating certain foods can alleviate these diseases.

Robin is a well-known chef who created Vibrant Cuisine, a fusion of international cuisines using antioxidant-rich ingredients to delight the palate and bring about wellness. For this book, she has developed meal plans and recipes that are as delicious as they are easy to follow. Those who adopt her plan can substantially lower their risk of most degenerative diseases.

This diet program is strict, and those who wish to follow it must be motivated to make a complete break from lifelong food habits. I believe that the effort is well worth it when one experiences the general improvement in well-being.

Richard Couey, PhD
Professor of Health Studies
Baylor University
Waco, TX 76798

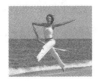

ACKNOWLEDGMENTS

First, I must acknowledge the Creator for this generous message of healing and wholeness. Second, I must thank my mother and father, Patty and Bob Jeep. Because of them, preparing healthy food became my life's calling. They were my greatest fans while I whirled concoctions in the blender and monopolized the family kitchen testing recipes.

My daughter, Alexandra Hohenlohe, has been endless in her encouragement and excitement by spreading the word throughout France where she lives. Thanks, also, to my brilliant and creative sister, Elisabeth Jeep, who helped me develop this idea into a business. She has been a never-ending source of encouragement as well as a great researcher.

I especially want to acknowledge my dearest friend, Aleka Zichy, who adopted the antioxidant style of eating from the beginning. She continually shares her creative wisdom with me and never ceases spreading information about the antioxidant lifestyle to everyone she knows in Europe, where she makes her home.

I am grateful to my former employers, who gave me the needed impetus to make this book happen.

And many thanks to the calm and steady support of my publisher Bob Friedman who immediately recognized the value of publishing this information. Also thanks to Joan Allen for providing her support and editing skills on seemingly endless days of frustration.

This book would not have its warmth without the talent and dedication of my friend Sherie Ellington who painstakingly reworked my words to make them flow with ease and grace. Thank you, also, to my life coach Ingrid Martine for helping me overcome self-imposed obstacles so I might also flow with ease and grace.

This book is only possible because of all the people who supported, encouraged, and helped me along the way. I would like to acknowledge some of them by name: Loy Burgess, Bob Phillips, Janet Bass, Greg Hochman, Lydia and Craig Hoffman, Fran Cincotti, Katya Pendill, Alexander Pashkowsky, Jim Wien, Chris Corsbie, Sara Wood, Jacquelyn Garcia, Darlene Youtes, Isabell Kelly, Lisa Torgersen, Karrie Priest, Renee Swann, Lisa Brazwell, and Jay Ehret.

Finally, I want to acknowledge Joel Fuhrman, MD, for his dedication in pursuing nutritional healing. I am very grateful to him for guiding me back to health after my riding accident. Joel and his wife Lisa supported me through many frustrating and painful days while I recovered.

Later, I worked in Joel's health clinic and watched many others overcome disease. Through this experience, my understanding of nutrition and its effect on health became even clearer. I will always be grateful to Joel and Lisa Fuhrman for letting me be part of their lives.

INTRODUCTION

In the good old days—before cities lured us off the farm—we had local roots, strong muscles, and simple diets. Our foods were rich with nutrients, our cattle grazed on the range, and natural fertilizers were used in the fields.

Today we are a society of packaged foods and drive-through windows. Our food is mass-produced, processed, preserved, and highly refined. As a result, less than 20 percent of calories (compared to 40 percent in 1900) in the Standard American Diet (SAD) come from fresh fruit, fresh vegetables, and whole grains.

According to studies that compare diet and disease profiles, SAD is associated with high rates of heart disease, hypertension, diabetes, and cancers of the breast, stomach, and colon, to name a few. In the United States, these diseases are at epidemic levels, but the body's ability to heal itself is amazing when given a nurturing environment.

The purpose of *The Super Antioxidant Diet* is to provide you with the facts and tools to help you achieve optimal health. If you need to lose weight, you will find that weight loss is another benefit of this diet.

This book is about far more than the healing properties of antioxidants. It is a holistic guide to creating a positive, nurturing lifestyle—dietary, spiritual, emotional, mental, and physical. The chapters are brief and the recipes are convenient and easy to prepare. We've even added a section on nutrition for your dog.

We hope you enjoy the journey to better health, and we hope you'll share your story with us at www.vibrantcuisine.com.

WHAT MAKES THE SUPER ANTIOXIDANT DIET UNIQUE AND SUCCESSFUL?

The Super Antioxidant Diet is an optimal eating plan based on medical principles and scientific studies.

Three sections are included in the book: Reclaim Your Health, Vibrant Cuisine, and Journey to Wholeness. In addition, Dr. Couey's simple yet effective exercise program entitled Just Move! is included as an appendix.

Trained chef Robin Jeep, who also shares her own personal journey to health using these eating techniques, developed the delicious Vibrant Cuisine recipes presented in this book.

What makes this plan successful? This diet is not about restriction but about developing healthy lifestyles and eating delicious food. Because Robin recognizes that people need choices, she has developed four separate diet plans—Fish Eaters, Meat and Fish Eaters, Ultimate Vegan, and Anti-Inflammation.

This book also contains the tools to overcome the Seven Primary Obstacles of transitioning into a healthier lifestyle, including:

Confusion • Doubt
Food Cravings • Digestive
Disturbances • Detoxification
Comfort • Peer Pressure

PART I

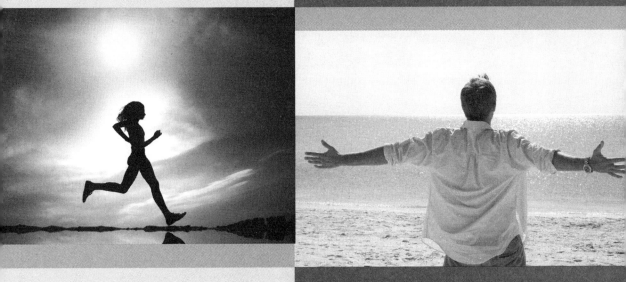

RECLAIM YOUR HEALTH

CHAPTER ONE

JOURNEY TO HELL AND BACK

Let me begin by sharing my own journey toward optimal health. The Super Antioxidant program has allowed me to heal from numerous conditions: bipolar disorder, dyslexia, irritable bowel syndrome (IBS), migraine headaches, hormone imbalances, skin disorders, prescription drug use, and major physical injuries caused by a horseback-riding accident. I believe my professional and personal experiences, coupled with Dr. Couey's guidance and oversight, qualify me to present you with this Super Antioxidant plan for healthy living.

A diet rich in antioxidants has only been part of my healing. My reconnection with my Creator has put me on the path to emotional and spiritual wholeness.

Getting to this point has not been easy. It has been a long road that goes all the way back to my conception. I always thought that my robust twin brother must have claimed most of the nutrients inside my mother's womb because he was much larger at birth and grew into a healthy, intelligent, good-looking, and very popular young man. In contrast, I became a dark-haired, scrawny, sickly, average, and unpopular child. In other words, I easily slipped into the role of the *consummate* victim.

I felt alone and lonely, but found I was connected to horses. My father was a rancher, so we always had horses. I began riding at age four.

I also found solace in my mother's brilliant cooking. Our home life revolved around the kitchen and her gourmet dinners. At times, she would even prepare international-themed dinners that spawned my interest in world cuisines.

Mother's expert skills and appreciation for good food came from my grandmother who grew up in Europe and studied at the famous Fanny Farmer Cooking School in New York City. Coincidentally, one of Farmer's quotes from *The Boston Cooking-School Cook*

Book seemed prophetic for my life and the age in which we now live:

> I certainly feel that the time is not far distant when knowledge of the principles of diet will be an essential part of one's education. Then mankind will eat to live, will be able to do better mental and physical work, and disease will be less frequent.

At eighteen, my life came to a terrible halt. My twin brother was murdered, senselessly—shot in the head at gunpoint. No one in the family knew what to do or how to cope. I immediately realized I had to search for personal meaning. At twenty, and with only $35 in my pocket, I jumped on a plane and flew to Europe.

I soon moved to Vienna, Austria, where my thinness was valued and I became a successful model. I found myself surrounded by an aristocratic crowd, and before I knew it, I was married to an Austrian prince.

My life in Austria afforded me the opportunity to learn the techniques and recipes from the private chefs who worked for my husband's family and others in our circle. As I developed and began eating the super antioxidant way, my slightly overweight husband did, too.

He became slender and his nagging skin problems disappeared. He also became more energetic and began running, something unheard of at that time in Vienna. During that period, I also met a racehorse owner and began training as a steeplechase jockey.

In the late 1970s, most successful models were extremely thin. I knew my modeling career required me to stay thin, but I was determined to remain healthy and strong as well. Riding horses, I learned, was one way to build endurance and gain strength. Eating green vegetables, fresh fruits, and nuts, I also learned, was the best way to keep strong and thin.

I tried to hide my insecurity and pain behind a glamorous model/actress/princess facade. Quite frankly, I was denying the emotional pain of my childhood and the loss of my brother. The pain was overwhelming. My lifestyle had become too fast-paced, undisciplined, and often unhealthy.

My tolerant husband and his family were subjected to my confused and rebellious behavior. My husband and I moved to New York City so that he could study film at NYU. He also thought it would help me to get away from the pressures of his family in Vienna.

My troubles were magnified by the intense emotional climate of New York.

In the early 1980s, I convinced my husband to move with me to Texas, but that still wasn't the answer. My emotional pain continued to drive me deeper into self-destruction.

Emotional problems finally destroyed my marriage. Physical problems ended my steeplechase career. It was during this time I was diagnosed with manic-depression (bipolar disorder). The feeling of failure and loss, as well as the stigma of mental illness, fed into my mindset of *victim*. But I still wouldn't acknowledge that my choices were negative and self-fulfilling. Fortunately, I was blessed with a higher power that allowed me to function and work.

By my late twenties, the headaches that had tortured me throughout my life developed into excruciating migraines. My energy level dropped drastically, and I was incapacitated with migraines, so fierce at times that I had to receive Imitrex (sumatriptan succinate) injections.

Horrible PMS all but crippled me in my thirties. My overall ability to reason was diminished by drug use: lithium, antidepressants, prescription painkillers, over-the-counter painkillers, and mood stabilizers.

When I was thirty-one, I had a spiritual awakening and began the slow process of finding my way to a healthy lifestyle—body, mind, and spirit. Because I was quite knowledgeable about nutrition and healthy eating, I landed a job at Whole Foods Market in the late 1980s. There I learned more about the healing effects of nutrients, herbs, and organic supplements. As a private chef, I began designing recipes and meal plans based on healthy eating.

In 1998, I began experiencing horrible abdominal pains. My doctor told me I had uterine fibroid tumors and needed a hysterectomy. I joyfully jumped at this relief. The doctor discovered a benign fibroid tumor the size of a honeydew melon during the surgery. I was relieved to know I wasn't crazy, that there was an explanation for the intense pain I had endured. After the surgery, however, I was given additional drugs to add to my already long list of pharmaceuticals.

During those difficult years, I flip-flopped between a dairy-rich vegetarian diet, a vegan diet, and a rich meat diet. I had grown to love the richest cheeses, best cappuccino, and finest wines, but I seldom consumed fruit because I had always thought it too high in calories. Instead, I ate primarily a meager-portioned, high-protein, low-carbohydrate diet to keep from gaining weight.

In my forties, a position as a private chef led me from Texas to Los Angeles. In LA, I was diagnosed with irritable bowel syndrome (IBS) and was prescribed the mild tranquilizer Librax (chlordiazepoxide and clidinium). At that point, I was already taking lithium, Neurontin (gabapentin; mood stabilizer), Imitrex, painkillers, and synthetic hormones. I didn't want to add more medications, although almost everyone I knew in LA was taking several medications. I just accepted it as part of life.

Like almost everyone in Hollywood, I began working on a film project—a young adult fantasy book that was to be animated. A major production company had shown interest in the film, but my mental abilities had become so diminished that I was unable to follow through. It was at that moment I realized my life had to change. *I had to change!*

One day, I met a fascinating woman with the clearest eyes I had ever seen. She was sharp and focused and her spiritual faith was something I had never witnessed before. As we became friends, she shared how a nutrient-dense vegan diet, and even "fasting," had cleansed her life. Her own personal struggles, she said, had led her to a deep spiritual faith and a vegan way of eating. She was the picture of health—and she actually practiced what she preached. I trusted her and began following her diet.

After two months of feeling rejuvenated, I was persuaded to wean myself off medication. I was very scared, but she assured me I would be just fine. I consulted my physician and slowly began tapering off the lithium and Neurontin. I felt great, unbelievably great. I also found that following a healthy diet changed my health and my entire outlook on life.

Although my mood swings have never returned, I never would have done anything so drastic without a doctor's guidance. I cannot emphasize this enough: No one should ever stop taking medication without the supervision of a supportive medical doctor.

Fast forward.

It was not until 2002 that I realized sharing this knowledge was my calling in life. I suffered a near-death experience when a horse I was riding fell on top of me. While in the trauma unit the doctors had little hope for me. I was severely hemorrhaging and had fractured fourteen pelvic bones, my sacrum, and both hips. Later, the doctors attributed my amazing and rapid recovery to a healthy lifestyle and nutrient-rich diet.

About a year after my accident, I began working as a private chef for a couple who owned three residences in the United States and one on a Caribbean island. I felt like my whole world revolved around packing, unpacking, and cooking. My digestive problems returned.

One day, my boss gave me a book on diet and nutrition, *Eat to Live,* by Joel Fuhrman, MD. As I began reading the book, everything I'd learned about dieting and nutrition—from my own steeplechase/modeling diet to the diet the woman in California had shared with me—made sense. Foods rich in nutrients are the foundation of vibrant health. Although I had always had the knowledge, I had not always eaten that way. Had I been consistent, I would have avoided some of the health problems I had endured for so long: mood swings, migraines, insomnia, hormonal problems, joint pain, digestive problems . . .

During my recovery period, I realized I had a gift to offer—one of hope and healing. This gift includes creating delicious and simply prepared dishes from antioxidant-rich foods. I teamed up with Dr. Couey, and we developed a healthy and delicious dietary program based on scientific principals. This program offers a holistic approach to nutritional education, personal growth, culinary instruction, physical fitness, and healthy social interaction.

At that point, I realized why God had put me around food all my life. I had always been successful in the food business—as a caterer, a Whole Foods marketing director, and a private chef. Things just never flowed smoothly in my attempts at other careers.

With the help of my sister, I set up the website www.vibrantcuisine.com. I also began working as a dietary assistant for Joel Fuhrman, MD, teaching cooking classes and providing support to his patients. Each life experience has added to my own personal journey toward wholeness. Now I am on a profound new journey to share this lifestyle with you. It is simply one more way I hope to fulfill God's direction for me to *Feed His Sheep.*

The amount of antioxidants that you maintain in your body is directly proportional to how long you will live.

—Richard Cutler, PhD, director of anti-aging research at National Institutes of Health[1]

ANTIOXIDANTS AND FREE RADICALS

Fruits and vegetables get their vibrant, rich colors from molecules called *antioxidants.* Antioxidants counteract the effect of *free radicals,* unstable electrons that alter the chemical structure of molecules.[2] Exposure to oxygen and sunlight, among other chemical stresses, produces the molecular reactions that form free radicals.

When we cut open an apple and expose it to the air, for instance, it turns brown. This browning process is caused by the production of free radicals that result from the fruit being exposed to the oxygen in the air. This process is known as *oxidative stress*.

As living, "breathing" creatures that need oxygen and sunlight to survive, we cannot avoid free radicals. On the other hand, uncontrolled free radical production can lead to a host of ailments, including cancer, arthritis, premature aging, and a general deterioration of health.

When we eat an abundance of fruits and vegetables, we benefit from the antioxidants in them. Their antioxidants actually protect us from the damaging effects of free radicals. This is the only way to be protected and to effectively minimize the chances of developing degenerative diseases.[3,4]

• The benefits of antioxidants are documented and proven. Antioxidant foods have become popular both in the news and on the shelves. Antioxidants have even won their own rating. The Oxygen Radical Absorbance Capacity (ORAC) rating is an analysis that measures the total antioxidant power of foods and other substances. These ratings have recently been included on the food labels of various food products.

• Antioxidants are best when consumed in their most natural form—vegetables, fruits, beans, nuts, and seeds. After all, God first created us to live on fresh, natural foods. In Genesis 1:29, He spoke these words: "Behold, I have given you every plant yielding seed that is on the surface of all the earth, and every tree which has fruit yielding seed; it shall be food for you . . ." How could we possibly improve upon His perfect plan?

• Optimal health can only be attained and maintained by eating an abundance and variety of plant foods. The word "plant" in the original Hebrew is Esab, "juicy stemmed plants." Today these plants would include a long list of fresh food: lettuce, chard, kale, spinach, and herbs, to name a few. These foods are all high in antioxidants.

• Science is now validating the ancient instruction of consuming high-nutrient, low-calorie foods. The writers of the Bible somehow knew that a variety of fresh foods was important for our health. And every day, new scientific studies are confirming that following this ancient instruction is the only way humans are able to nourish their cells sufficiently to avoid degenerative diseases. In the Western world, the history of these disciplines goes back to the early nineteenth century in Europe. In the late 1980s, science began to hone in on nutrition and the cell. The results of this scientific research are validating what the people who practiced these healing disciplines intuitively knew.[5,6,7] Naturopathic doctors have been advocating this type of diet for some time. Medical doctors are now beginning to recognize the importance of this type of dietary plan.

• Because antioxidant-rich foods tend to be lower in calories, they are a natural way to lose and/or maintain a healthy weight. Even though the Super Antioxidant Diet offers an abundance of food, maintaining a healthy weight is just one of its benefits. Studies on lower calorie diets that contain an abundance of antioxidant-rich foods have shown that such diets are effective in increasing health and longevity.

• A low-calorie diet can actually benefit our health. Studies show that restrictive diets have a powerful effect on our ability to protect against atherosclerosis, a condition caused by fatty material clogging up arterial walls. Arteries are blood vessels that carry oxygen from the heart to other parts of the body. With these types of diets, glucose, inflammation, and triglyceride levels typically decrease. With all of this proof, why aren't more people eating a well-balanced, high-nutrient, low-calorie diet? Have we been conditioned by advertising, peer pressure, personal habit, and a fast-food lifestyle to simply turn away from the facts? Have we become so complacent that we've ignored our health? Just look around! We can no longer ignore the physical, emotional, psychological, and financial effects of being unhealthy. The Super Antioxidant Diet is all about health, vitality, abundance, and experiencing the inner joy for which we were designed. With this program:

• You will not focus on calories, portion control, or deprivation. Change that mindset! Diets based on limited portions go against human nature. It's no wonder people fail. The primary goal of this eating program is to keep your body full of antioxidant foods, just as nature intended. You will be required to eat a lot of food!

• You don't have to become a nutritional expert to be successful at this program. You won't have to take a class, but you will learn about foods that contain the most antioxidants. You will also learn how to combine these foods into delicious recipes. In addition, you'll learn how to prepare your kitchen, how to shop, and how to stay committed to your plan while traveling and eating out.

• You will increase your ability to achieve your health goal. Whether your goal is to lose weight, gain more energy, or modify the effects of illness or disease, don't forget to see your physician first. Then get regular checkups to document your progress.

• You won't have to follow any off-the-wall, unscientific procedure to cleanse your body of free radicals. In fact, if you follow this program, you will be eating mounds of fresh tasty foods while developing an optimistic mindset.

• You aren't expected to be perfect. This eating plan does require changing habits, but it is equally important to be flexible and spontaneous. Don't set yourself up to fail. Look at this eating plan as a pair of training wheels preparing you for the journey toward lifelong wellness. Recognize that change takes practice and time. And every accomplishment, big or small, counts. There is a reason you are reading this book. Perhaps you have decided to take that courageous first step to change your future—a change that will lead you to a better quality of life. Perhaps you are now ready to become empowered with the tools of healthy, abundant living.

SELF-ASSESSMENT

Self-knowledge is the beginning of self-improvement.
—Baltasar Gracián (1601–1658)

Optimal health is not all about diet and weight. It is the combination of a healthy heart, soul, body, and mind—and it results from the peaceful positive sense of being that results from hard work and positive action. This Bible verse sums it *all* up: "For where your treasure is, there also is your heart" (Matthew 6:21).

The following questionnaire may help you identify areas in your life that potentially impede you from achieving optimal health.

You have some work to do if you answered yes to any of these questions, but don't be quick to throw them away. They will serve as a reference point on your journey to optimal health.

After you begin this journey, glance at your answers and note any positive changes you are experiencing because of your altered behavior. Don't be too hard on yourself. Remember, you will not have to be perfect and your physical or emotional problems won't suddenly disappear. Change is a process, and reversing the longtime effects of negative behavior can take a while. By following the Super Antioxidant Diet, however,

SELF-ASSESSMENT QUESTIONNAIRE   DATE _____

1. Do you take medications? (If yes, list your medications and dosage, how long you have taken these medications, and why you take them.)

2. Do you experience restless sleep or insomnia? If yes, how often per week?

3. Do you suffer from bowel problems such as constipation, diarrhea, or irregular bowel movements? If so, how often per week?

4. Do you suffer from indigestion or acid reflux? If so, how often per week? What time of day?

5. Is your blood pressure outside of normal range?

6. Are your blood cholesterol and LDL outside of the normal range?

7. Do you suffer from allergies? If yes, list your allergies.

8. Do you have food cravings? If so, for what? How often?

9. Do you binge eat? If so, how often?

10. Do you have headaches or migraines? If so, when? How often?

11. Do you suffer from body aches? What kind?

12. Do you often catch a cold or the flu?

13. Do you struggle to accomplish daily tasks?

14. Do you lack the time and/or energy to participate in regular recreation? (If no, list the type of activities you do. How often do you participate in them?)

15. Do you lack a solid network of family and friends that provide you with honest, emotional support?

16. Do you easily become restless, bored, or frustrated?

17. Are you often irritated, frustrated, or tired?

18. Are you often sad or depressed?

19. Do you sometimes wonder if you will ever be able to relax, enjoy life, and/or have fun?

BMI CHART

To find your BMI, locate your height in the left-hand column and your weight in the correct right-hand column. Based on where the two meet, you will find your BMI number in the top row.

WEIGHT _____   HEIGHT _____   BMI _____

BMI	19	20	21	22	23	24	25	26	27	28	29	30	31	32	33	34	35
4'10" (58")	91	96	100	105	110	115	119	124	129	134	138	143	148	153	158	162	167
4'11" (59")	94	99	104	109	114	119	124	128	133	138	143	148	153	158	163	168	173
5' (60")	97	102	107	112	118	123	128	133	138	143	148	153	158	163	168	174	179
5'1" (61")	100	106	111	116	122	127	132	137	143	148	153	158	164	169	174	180	185
5'2" (62")	104	109	115	120	126	131	136	142	147	153	158	164	169	175	180	186	191
5'3" (63")	107	113	118	124	130	135	141	146	152	158	163	169	175	180	186	191	197
5'4" (64")	110	116	122	128	134	140	145	151	157	163	169	174	180	186	192	197	204
5'5" (65")	114	120	126	132	138	144	150	156	162	168	174	180	186	192	198	204	210
5'6" (66")	118	124	130	136	142	148	155	161	167	173	179	186	192	198	204	210	216
5'7" (67")	121	127	134	140	146	153	159	166	172	178	185	191	198	204	211	217	223
5'8" (68")	125	131	138	144	151	158	164	171	177	184	190	197	203	210	216	223	230
5'9" (69")	128	135	142	149	155	162	169	176	182	189	196	203	209	216	223	230	236
5'10" (70")	132	139	146	153	160	167	174	181	188	195	202	209	216	222	229	236	243
5'11" (71")	136	143	150	157	165	172	179	186	193	200	208	215	222	229	236	243	250
6' (72")	140	147	154	162	169	177	184	191	199	206	213	221	228	235	242	250	258
6'1" (73")	144	151	159	166	174	182	189	197	204	212	219	227	235	242	250	257	265
6'2" (74")	148	155	163	171	179	186	194	202	210	218	225	233	241	249	256	264	272
6'3' (75")	152	160	168	176	184	192	200	208	216	224	232	240	248	256	264	272	279

Source: Evidence Report of Clinical Guidelines on the Identification, Evaluation, and Treatment of Overweight and Obesity in Adults, 1998. NIH/National Heart, Lung, and Blood Institute (NHLBI), Centers for Disease Control and Prevention, United States Department of Health and Human Services

UNDERSTANDING YOUR BMI (WOMEN AND MEN)

BMI less than 18.5 may indicate underweight • BMI 19–25 healthy range
BMI 25–30 indicates overweight • BMI above 30 indicates obesity

you will be better equipped with the tools to reduce and possibly eliminate those bothersome "yes" answers from your life.

YOUR IDEAL WEIGHT

Now comes the difficult part for many people. The journey to optimal health begins with maintaining a healthy weight.

The body mass index (BMI) is commonly used to help determine if a person is overweight and at risk for health problems. According to the Centers for Disease Control and Prevention, the correlation between the BMI number and body fatness is fairly strong; however, the correlation varies by sex, race, and age. These variations include the following examples:[8,9]

- At the same BMI, women tend to have more body fat than men.

- At the same BMI, older people, on average, tend to have more body fat than younger adults.

- Highly trained athletes may have a high BMI because of increased muscularity rather than increased body fatness.

It is also important to remember that BMI is only one factor related to risk for disease. For assessing someone's likelihood of developing overweight or obesity-related diseases, the National Heart, Lung, and Blood Institute guidelines recommend looking at two other predictors:

- waist circumference (because abdominal fat is a predictor of risk for obesity-related diseases)

- diseases and conditions associated with obesity (for example, high blood pressure or physical inactivity)

CHAPTER TWO

DIETARY GUIDELINES

BACKGROUND

Humans and apes, especially chimpanzees, are similar in physical and genetic design. Unlike other mammals, man and ape are built with long, pouched colons and short, blunt teeth to accommodate a natural diet of plants. Although both species are physically *able* to digest flesh, excessive consumption causes a host of health problems.

A radical experiment developed by a nutritionist from King's College Hospital illustrates this point very well.[1] He designed an eating regimen based on the natural diet of apes. The diet generously provided the daily nutritional requirements and approximately 2,000 calories for the women and 2,300 calories for the men. The nutritionist hoped to confirm that plant foods could actually lower cholesterol and blood pressure level.

Nine volunteers, aged thirty-six to forty-nine, moved into an enclosed area next to the ape house at Paignton Zoo in Devon, England. For twelve days, they consumed up to five kilos (eleven pounds) of raw antioxidant rich vegetables, fruits, and nuts. Other than including oily fish to ensure an adequate intake of fatty acids essential to human health, the diet was that of their fellow primates.

At the conclusion of the experiment, the cholesterol levels of the volunteers had dropped an average of 23 percent, blood pressure levels had lowered to an average of 122/76, and the group lost an average of more than a whopping nine pounds.

As you can imagine, eleven pounds of food is a lot of food! Eleven pounds of raw plant food is also a lot of fiber to someone accustomed to eating a low-fiber diet. Not surprisingly, most of the volunteers were unable to eat all of their daily rations. Most of us need to consume at least 1,700 to 2,400 calories and at least forty grams of protein per day. A very small woman might only need to consume 1,500 calories, or an endurance athlete would need more than 2,400.

In order to obtain sixty calories and seven grams of protein from lettuce, you'd have to eat a pound of it. By consuming a pound of broccoli, you'd only receive seventy-eight calories of energy and eight grams of protein. Kale, on the other hand, contains 227 calories and fifteen grams of protein per pound.

Although plant foods are naturally lower in calories and density, it is unnecessary to eat eleven pounds of raw plant foods to receive daily health requirements. You will learn, however, that on the Super Antioxidant Diet, you will be encouraged to eat very generous portions.

RAW FOOD DIETS:
Know the Facts!

I am including this section to discourage those wanting to jump into a diet consisting entirely of raw plant foods. A person would need to consume approximately four to five pounds of produce each day (which equals about fifty to sixty grams of fiber) to receive the nutrients needed to be healthy. On a good day, the average American consumes around nineteen grams of fiber. It's not beneficial

to suddenly load the digestive tract with almost three times that much!

The following chart will give you an idea of how much raw produce a person must consume to ingest enough nutrients to avoid deficiency. It totals four to five pounds of fresh produce and equals five fresh fruits and two huge dinner plates loaded with salad. Even if a person were able to consume that much raw produce, a digestive tract that is not accustomed to this type of diet may not be able to absorb the necessary nutrients. While I worked for Dr. Fuhrman, I learned about many patients on raw food diets that were suffering from nutritional deficiencies.

Do wolves ponder over what diet to eat—or whales, or bears? Of course not! Humans are the only species that believe in choosing diets according to preference—low carb, low glycemic, high protein, blood type, body type, all-raw foods, and so on.

Numerous scientific studies have concluded that only one basic diet plan is optimal for the human species—a diet plan high in antioxidant foods. The Super Antioxidant Diet goes even further by illustrating how super antioxidant health may also be achieved by eating a variety of delicious dishes.

The diet also includes information based on individual needs and requirements. For

DAILY RAW FOOD INTAKE

½ pound romaine lettuce • 2 stalks celery • ¼ pound kale leaves • ⅔ cup sprouted kidney beans • 1 pear • 1 medium Roma tomato • ½ cup raw cashews • 1 orange • ¼ onion • ½ cup sunflower seeds • 1 kiwi fruit • ¼ pound cabbage • 1 tablespoon nutritional yeast • 1 banana • ¼ pound bok choy • 2 tablespoons tahini • 1 cup blueberries • ⅓ pound broccoli 3 teaspoons cider vinegar • ½ cucumber • ½ medium avocado • 1 clove garlic

NUTRITIONAL BREAKDOWN

Calories	1973
% Calories from fat	42.6%
% Calories from carbohydrates	44.6%
Calories from protein	12.8%
Total fat	102g RDA 157%
Saturated fat	17g RDA 85%
Monounsaturated fat	48g RDA 217%
Polyunsaturated fat	27g RDA 123%
Cholesterol	0mg RDA 0%
Total carbohydrates	240g RDA 80%
Dietary fiber	58g RDA 232%
Sodium	382mg RDA 76%
Folacin	1313mcg RDA 328%
Protein	69g RDA 138%
Potassium	6690mg RDA 191%
Calcium	912mg RDA 91%
Iron	28mg RDA 154%
Zinc	15mg RDA 99%
Vitamin C	603mg RDA 1005%
Vitamin A	44744IU RDA 895%
Vitamin B-6	3.6mg RDA 180%
Vitamin B-12	0mcg RDA 0%
Thiamin B-1	3.8mg RDA 250%
Riboflavin B-2	1.8mg RDA 107%
Niacin	17mg RDA 86%

instance, an athlete will require more calories and protein than a non-athlete. A diabetic person will need to eat in a particular way until glucose levels are stabilized within the normal range.

Nonetheless, a certain amount of nutrients are needed to build strong, healthy cells. Our bodies are always replacing cells. Healthy foods will build healthier new cells and replace inferior ones. Organs *regenerate* rather than *degenerate*. As cells and arteries become healthier, blood flows more freely throughout the body and the mind becomes clear. With mental clarity, thinking becomes more optimistic and positive cycles replace the negative ones.

SUPER ANTIOXIDANT GUIDELINES

Many people transition into the Super Antioxidant Diet without any discomfort. Others, especially ones used to eating a low-fiber diet, experience stronger reactions such as gas, colon cramping, and diarrhea. If you experience any discomfort, try eating easier-to-digest foods at first—foods like steamed zucchini, winter squashes, sweet potatoes, tofu, and a small amount of fish and chicken. As your digestive tract settles down, you will be able to introduce more raw vegetables, but it may take from six weeks to three months.

Here are some additional suggestions:

• Use commonsense servings. Allow differences in body size, activity level, and age.

• Consume organically raised foods whenever possible, although most non-organic items work just fine. I indicate the few items that should only be consumed if organic because of residual pesticides and fungicides. *Look for the (O) next to these items.*

• Avoid or limit high-glycemic fruits (bananas, watermelons, pineapples, kiwis, and mangos) if you are trying to lose weight or are being medically supervised to lower blood sugar through nutritional means. *Look for the (A) next to these items.*

VEGETABLES

The famous Jack LaLanne said in an interview that he eats at least ten different vegetables per day. It sounds daunting, but you should aim for that as well! And combining both raw and cooked vegetables into your diet is the best way.

Suggested daily intake:

• One pound or three to five cups of fresh salad including a variety of raw vegetables

• Three cups of a variety of cooked vegetables. There is no limit on leafy green and colored vegetables.

Artichokes • Asparagus • Baby Bok Choy • Bamboo Shoots Beets (O) • Bell Peppers Belgian Endive Leaves • Bok Choy • Broccoli • Broccoli Sprouts • Brussels Sprouts Cabbage • Carrots (O) Cauliflower • Celery (O) Chard • Corn (O) • Cucumber Eggplant • Fennel Root • Green Beans • Green Peas • Greens (all types) • Kale • Kohlrabi Mushrooms • Okra • Onions (O) Parsley • Peppers • Radishes Snow Peas • Spinach (O) String Beans • Sugar Snap Peas Summer Squash • Tomatoes Turnips (O) • Water Chestnuts Zucchini

Note: Eating raw kale can be tough on the digestive system. Until your body has adapted to raw vegetables, steam and chop kale prior to eating.

FRESH FRUIT

Recommended daily intake: Four to five servings of different fresh or frozen fruits/berries. (A serving is half a cup of high-glycemic fruits *or* one cup of low-glycemic fruits or berries.)

Nonorganic Acceptable

Blackberries • Blueberries Grapefruits • Melons Oranges • Papayas • Pears Persimmons • Plums • Prunes Tangerines • Organic Only Apples (O) • Apricots (O) Cantaloupes (O) • Grapes (O) Strawberries (O) • Raspberries (O) Nectarines (O) • Peaches (O)

Avoid (if medically necessary)

Bananas (A) • Kiwis (A) Mangoes (A) • Pineapples (A) Watermelons (A)

COOKED LEGUMES

Recommended daily intake: One to two cups of cooked legumes *or* a half-cup serving of legumes with fish or meat.

Black Beans • Black-Eyed Peas
Cannellini Beans • Fava Beans
Garbanzo Beans • Lentils
Lima Beans • Navy Beans
Pinto Beans • Red Kidney
Beans • Soybeans

Note: When raw legumes are properly soaked and germinated, their nutritive value increases, usually to levels equal to or exceeding those of the cooked bean.[2] Some people have problems digesting raw sprouted legumes, and there is some controversy about raw legumes containing certain toxic chemicals. Blending raw foods into dips, smoothies, and gazpachos is important because it breaks down the plant foods' cellular walls, greatly increasing nutrient absorption.

STARCHY VEGETABLES

Recommended daily intake: One to three half-cup servings cooked, unless you are trying to lose weight (limit to none or one serving per day) or needing to lower blood sugar (avoid altogether).

Carrots • Chestnuts • Corn

Parsnips (O if possible)
Pumpkins • Sweet Potatoes (O if possible) • Turnips (O if possible)
White Potatoes (sparingly)
Winter Squash

Note: White potatoes cause glucose levels to rise, which results in increased insulin production. Insulin affects the enzymes that produce inflammatory arachidonic acid.

WHOLE GRAINS

Recommended daily intake: One to three servings per day, unless you are trying to lose weight (then limit to no more than a half-cup cooked whole grains per day or one slice of bread or omit completely), are athletic, or are trying to gain weight (increase daily servings accordingly).

Barley • Millet • Oatmeal
Polenta • Quinoa • Wheat
berries • Whole-grain breads
Whole-grain rice

Note: Breads on grocery shelves are often not healthful, although their labels might deceive you. Purchase your bread from a health food store but make sure its ingredients don't include chemical preservatives or high fructose corn syrup. An excellent alternative is Ezekiel 4:9 Organic Sprouted Whole Grain Products from Food for Life (FFL; www.foodforlife.com). According to the website, FFL's Organic Sprouted Whole Grain Products are inspired by the Holy Scripture verse:

Take also unto thee Wheat, and Barley, and Beans, and Lentils, and Millet, and Spelt, and put them in one vessel, and make bread of it . . . (Ezekiel 4:9)

ANTIOXIDANT HIGH-FAT PLANT FOODS
Raw Nuts and Seeds

Consuming good fat is both healthy and important. By eating healthy fat only available in whole foods, you increase your intake of antioxidants. Your goal is to limit other types of oil. After all, think about how many olives, vegetables, or nuts you would have to eat to get one teaspoon of oil.

Recommended daily intake:

Raw Nuts and Seeds: 12 raw nuts per day or 2 tablespoons raw seeds. *If you find that you can't control your consumption of nuts, avoid them altogether until* you have changed your taste preferences. If you are eating dishes that contain nuts or nut butters, avoid extra nuts.

Avocados: ¼ to 1 whole small or medium avocado. *If trying to lose weight, keep your avocado consumption to no more than ¼ per day. If you have coronary problems, check with your cardiologist before eating avocados.*

ANIMAL PRODUCTS

Recommended daily intake if meat eater: moderate servings (fewer than 150 calories per day or no more than four ounces per day of lean meat, skinless poultry breast, wild game, wild fish, or skim milk or yogurt). Better yet, reduce it to fewer than 4 (3 to 4 ounces) servings per week.

MEAT AND DAIRY
Know the Facts!

In ancient times, people ate dairy and other animal products because they lived in harsh environments where fresh produce was not readily available. In religious rituals they sacrificed animals and often ate the flesh. Their livestock was naturally raised, unlike most of the meat sold for food on today's market. Even meats with labels like "free-range" are questionable.

Organically raised meat does not necessarily mean grass-fed or free-range. And the label "free-range" does not mean the animals always roam freely. In fact, animals don't have to leave the stall or coop to be labeled "free-range."

The USDA's ambiguous free-range standards only require that outdoor access be available for an unspecified time each day. Does that mean the access to open space is large or small? Is the access available for more than a few minutes per day? And how much space is given the animal while inside the coop or barn?

To find out if a meat is *truly* free-range, ask the manager of the meat department at your local grocery store. Better yet, purchase the products directly from the grower. If you are unable to locate or feel you can't afford truly free-range meat, eliminate meat altogether.

ARACHIDONIC ACID AND INFLAMMATION

Although the only healthy animal is one that can roam freely and graze at will, meat doesn't contain *any* antioxidants. And most poultry, beef, and lamb on today's farms are fed grains rather than a natural diet of grass. This "upset" in diet

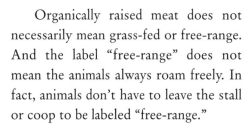

INFLAMMATORY DISEASES IN THE U.S.

Proven:
Asthma • Alzheimer's
Allergies • Arthritis • Gout
Lupus • Colitis • Crohn's Disease
Celiac Disease • Psoriasis

Strongly Suspected
Atherosclerosis • Diabetes
Nephritus • Hepatitus
Thyroiditis • Osteoarthritis
Bronchitis • Emphysema

Suspected
Alzheimer's • Cancer

causes an excess production of arachidonic acid.[3,4] Research has linked arachidonic acid to inflammatory diseases.[5] Arachidonic acid is also found in the fatty tissue of muscle meat, organ meats, and egg yolks. Our bodies also produce it when we have high insulin levels.

Arachidonic acid has been proven or suspected to cause and contribute to a long list of diseases.[6,7]

In chapter 6, Bare Minimum Supplements, we recommend a specifically formulated essential fatty acid supplement to help combat inflammation. All of the Super Antioxidant Diet meal plans are designed to fight inflammation as well, and the Ultimate Vegan and Anti-Inflammation plans especially so.

Excess animal protein upsets the pH balance of the body. Whereas plant foods are alkaline and calcium-rich, animal protein increases the production of metabolic acid. To neutralize this excess acid, calcium is leached from bones and excreted through the urine, decreasing bone density. Calcium in the urinary tract results in an increased risk for developing kidney stones.[8]

Some of the best antioxidant and calcium-rich foods include:

Bok choy • Turnip greens
Collard greens • Kale
Romaine lettuce • Tofu
Broccoli • Sesame seeds (ground)

Numerous studies reveal that dairy products, including cheese, are not healthy for children or adults. After all, cow's milk is designed to develop a calf from thirty pounds to four hundred pounds by the time it is weaned about six months later. Human beings are the only mammal species that continues to drink milk after being weaned.

Today, hormones and antibiotics are the order of the day on animal farms and these drugs can be found in the milk that's produced. Additionally, the primary component of milk protein in both nonfat and whole dairy called casein has been shown to promote some forms of cancer, at least in animals. One study, at Cornell University, revealed that casein tends to promote tumor growth. Casein has also been shown to increase coronary artery blockages in animals.

FISH
Know the Facts!

Fish does offer a healthy alternative to animal products, but it's wise to be cautious. Farm-raised fish tends to be high in arachidonic acid, and many types of fish contain high concentrations of mercury and other pollutants. Anchovies, herring, mackerel, and wild salmon actually help combat arachidonic acid. Wild salmon from less polluted waters such as Alaska are always the best choice as the fish contains a hefty portion of healthy omega-3 fatty acids.

Catfish, shellfish, and carp tend to accumulate more pollutants than other types of fish. And both catfish and shellfish live on the waste and toxins expelled from other fish.

Clams, oysters, mussels, and scallops are filter feeders. They get their food from filtering massive amounts of water.

These creatures consume whatever chemicals, toxins, bacteria, and viruses happen to be in the water where they live.

Almost all of the shrimp eaten in the United States is imported and more than 80 percent of that is farm raised. Most of these shrimp farms are found in Southeast Asia, where labor and environmental standards are less controlled than in the United States. These waters are often full of pesticides, antibiotics, and other chemicals.

If you like fish, we recommend eating a small serving (three to four ounces) of wild salmon three to four times a week. If you choose to eat shellfish of any kind, research its origin whenever possible.

If you eat meat, consume only small portions (three to four ounces two or three times per week) of lean free-range chicken breast, free-range turkey breast, lean wild game, and even less frequent and smaller portions of grass-fed beef or buffalo.

Fortunately, we are now blessed with an enormous variety of fresh and frozen produce throughout the year. The choice to eat animal products is a personal one. Here are the recommendations for consuming animal products.

Recommended:

- Anchovies, herring, mackerel, wild salmon

- Lean free-range chicken breast, free-range turkey breast

- Lean wild game

- Infrequent, small servings of grass-fed beef or buffalo

- Younger, smaller fish

Not recommended:

- Clams, oysters, mussels, shrimp, crayfish, lobster, squid, octopus, eel, scallops, catfish, carp

- Farm-raised fish of any type

- Grain-fed beef, poultry, or lamb

- Milk and milk products

- Egg yolks

- Pork

The dietary law found in the books of Leviticus and Deuteronomy in the Bible forbids the consumption of bottom-feeding fish. Today these guidelines are being recommended and validated by scientific studies.

SUPER HEROES:
Cruciferous Vegetables

The flowering plants in the mustard and cabbage family belong to a group of vegetables called Cruciferae. Interestingly, this name is derived from four-petal flowers that resemble a crucifix.

These foods have astonished researchers with their amazing healing properties. Among other things, cruciferous vegetables contain potent antioxidants that are believed to be responsible for lowering the risk of certain types of cancer and other degenerative diseases.[9] Cruciferous vegetables also help reduce the risk of cardiovascular disease.

Combine whole, raw vegetables in a blender for a refreshing drink (and you'll also get the benefit of extra fiber), or consume raw cruciferous vegetables as just the fresh juice alone, or include them chopped in a salad.

ARUGULA

Arugula is high in vitamin A, vitamin C, and niacin. As with all leafy greens, it is highly alkaline. Its peppery tartness adds zest to any salad.

BROCCOLI

Broccoli contains the super antioxidant sulforaphane. Researchers at Johns Hopkins University School of Medicine discovered that sulforaphane stimulates natural detoxifying enzymes in the body.[10,11] It is also the most powerful natural inhibitor of tumor growth. Studies suggest that you need to eat about two pounds of broccoli or other cruciferous vegetables per week to cut your risk of cancer in half.

BROCCOLI SPROUTS

Broccoli sprouts contain a much higher concentration of sulforaphane than mature broccoli.[12] I recommend that you eat an ounce or two of broccoli sprouts every day. Look for the trade brand Brocco (www.broccosprouts.com) in your supermarket. These little sprouts are so high in antioxidants that Johns Hopkins University has a patent pending on them.

BRUSSELS SPROUTS

Studies have shown that Brussels sprouts detoxify aflatoxin, a fungus linked to cancer, particularly liver cancer. Aflatoxin has been found in peanuts, corn, and rice.

A diet high in Brussels sprouts has been shown to reduce DNA damage, which may also reduce cancer risks. In addition, Brussels sprouts contain an abundance of vitamin A and beta carotene, which play important roles in defense against infection and also promote healthy skin.

DAIKON

This large, elongated, white winter radish is esteemed for its medicinal properties and is often used in home remedies. Many Eastern health practitioners claim that daikon cleanses the blood, promotes energy circulation, and increases the metabolic rate. With regular consumption, it is reported to help prevent the common cold, flu, and respiratory infections.

CABBAGE

Cabbage is another potent anti-cancer food and has also been shown to effectively treat ulcers. In a study by Stanford University School of Medicine, raw cabbage juice was most beneficial for treating ulcers.

CAULIFLOWER

As with all cruciferous vegetables, cauliflower contains the compounds that stimulate natural defenses against carcinogens. The vegetable's white color is due to its leaves, which prevent it from developing chlorophyll. There are other varieties as well. The green variety contains more vitamins A and C than the white.

COLLARD GREENS

Collard greens, a member of the headless cabbage family, are an excellent source of calcium.

KALE

Kale leads the pack of cruciferous vegetables. Kale is extremely rich in absorbable calcium and carotenoid antioxidants, powerful cancer fighters.

Because cooking destroys some of its nutrients while optimizing the absorption of others, I recommend consuming both uncooked and cooked kale. Raw kale's insoluble fiber can be tough on the digestive system, so add it slowly to your diet.

Blending and/or juicing uncooked kale is a great way to get the antioxidants in the raw form. Juicing raw kale gives you the powerful nutrients without the hard-to-digest fiber.

KOHLRABI

Kohlrabi tastes a bit like a turnip and is excellent for indigestion. It is also a good source of fiber and contains high amounts of vitamin C, calcium, and potassium.

MUSTARD GREENS

Mustard greens contain high amounts of antioxidant nutrients. All varieties of greens have about the same nutrient density, although kale leads the group. You should include all of them in your diet for optimal health.

RADISHES

Radishes are said to stimulate the appetite and have diuretic properties. They are also recommended for colds, flu, and respiratory infections because they are high in vitamin C and bioflavonoids.

TURNIPS AND RUTABAGAS

Rutabagas are members of the turnip family. While buried in the earth, these root vegetables draw their nutrients directly from the soil.

WATERCRESS

Watercress is a peppery leafy green that grows in flowing spring waters. Found in most supermarkets, it makes a wonderful addition to fresh salad. In addition to tasting great, watercress is a potent source of isothiocyanates, the natural chemical that stimulates the breakdown of potential carcinogens. It is also a source of sulforaphane, the most powerful natural chemical for stopping tumor growth.

SUPERHERO SIDEKICKS

BEANS/LEGUMES

Beans provide an abundance of healing nutrients. Low-fat beans are high in folate, potassium, protein, and fiber. They also provide an excellent source of soluble fiber. As they pass through the digestive tract, they grab and trap bile that contains cholesterol, removing it before it can be absorbed. Numerous studies have shown that beans lower cholesterol, curb appetite, and help the body regulate insulin.[13,14]

In addition to the overall health benefits, certain compounds that are found in beans have been shown to inhibit healthy cells from turning cancerous and inhibit cancer cells from growing. A recently released study indicated that a higher intake of beans and lentils was associated with a considerably lower risk of breast cancer in women.

When cooked with beans, the sea vegetable kombu helps reduce flatulence while adding nutrients.

BERRIES

Berries are one of nature's most nutrient-dense gifts.[15] Cranberries and blueberries contain compounds that help prevent and eliminate bladder infections. Dark berries such as raspberries, strawberries, and blueberries have been shown to have anti-cancer properties. Research has even shown that their powerful antioxidants may slow down the aging process. Berries also contain lutein, which helps promote healthy vision.

CARROTS

Studies have shown that eating two uncooked carrots every other day provides enough beta-carotene to reduce stroke risk in men with symptoms of heart disease.

CHILI PEPPERS

Chili peppers contain the antioxidant capsaicin and have blood-thinning properties that help prevent strokes and lower cholesterol. Additionally, they help satisfy salt cravings.

CITRUS FRUITS

Citrus fruits are high in vitamin C and bioflavonoids. These two nutrients likely work together to produce a positive effect on the immune system.

GARLIC

Since ancient times, garlic has been used medicinally. Garlic has been credited with lowering cholesterol and blood pressure as well as helping fight infection. It may also contain chemicals that fight cancer.

GOJI BERRIES

Native to Asia, the goji berry is known as the longevity fruit and is one of the most antioxidant-rich plant foods known to man. Typically sun-dried and somewhat sweet and tart, goji berries are valued as food as well as for medicinal properties.

They contain eighteen amino acids, more beta carotene than carrots, more iron than spinach, and twenty-one trace minerals. They also contain vitamins B-1, B-2, B-6, E, and very high levels of C.

In Tibet, goji berries have been used for thousands of years to treat kidney and liver problems, eye problems, skin rashes, psoriasis, allergies, insomnia, diabetes, tuberculosis, and high blood pressure.

GREEN TEA

According to some studies, green tea may be useful for the treatment of arteriosclerosis, high cholesterol, certain cancers, irritable bowel syndrome (IBS), diabetes, liver disease, weight loss, and cognitive impairment. Other studies claim differently. Nonetheless, green tea contains the antioxidants that keep cells healthy, and many doctors give their cancer patients green tea capsules as part of treatment.

Because green tea does contain caffeine, I recommend no more than two cups per day.

MANGOS, KIWIS, PINEAPPLES, AND PAPAYAS

These fruits are rich in vitamin C and contain high amounts of enzymes and antioxidants. These nutrients help combat of a host of diseases such as autoimmune disorders, allergies, and cancer.

MUSHROOMS

Many types of mushrooms contain compounds that stimulate the immune system. Shitake, enoki, and reishi have been shown to have anti-cancer and antiviral effects.

POMEGRANATE SEEDS AND JUICE

Pomegranates are extremely high in some powerful antioxidants.[16,17] Add pomegranate to smoothies or drink a few ounces of juice per day.

SEA VEGETABLES

Sea vegetables, often referred to as seaweed, have been harvested and eaten for centuries. These vegetables are one of the richest sources of minerals, essentially fat-free, and very low in calories. They are rich in calcium, phosphorous, magnesium, iron, iodine, and sodium. Sea vegetables also have anti-inflammatory properties.

Some studies indicate that seaweed has the ability to inhibit the absorption of heavy metals and radioactive pollutants.

As mentioned earlier, the sea vegetable kombu helps reduce flatulence while adding nutrients when cooked with beans.

SOYBEANS AND TOFU

Studies have shown that people who regularly eat soy products have lower rates of prostate, colon, lung, rectal, and stomach cancers.

In the *Journal of the American College of Nutrition*, Kenneth D. R. Setchell, PhD, contradicted earlier reports discouraging women with breast cancer from eating soy. He stated: "[R]ecommendations to avoid soy foods, now being given by many health professionals to these patients, are not based on any clinical evidence to support this advice."[18]

SPINACH

Spinach contains vitamins and minerals that help control the spread of cancer. These nutrients can reduce the risk of heart disease, stroke, and osteoporosis.

TOMATOES

Lycopenes, antioxidants found in tomatoes, have been reported to decrease the risk of prostate cancer. Lycopenes are more absorbable when cooked.

FOOD DIARY

The food diary on page 30 serves as a guide that will help you chart the estimated amounts of Super Antioxidant foods you are eating and identify areas where you may be lacking. Make copies to chart additional weeks.

FOOD DIARY DATE _____

FOOD	DAY						
	1	2	3	4	5	6	7
RAW VEGETABLES 2 to 3 servings or one (1) large Salad							
COOKED VEGETABLES 3 servings							
CRUCIFEROUS VEGETABLES 1 serving							
COOKED LEGUMES ½ to 1 serving							
FRUIT 3 to 5 servings							
BLUEBERRIES 1 cup							
STARCHY VEGETABLES 1 serving (limit or avoid to increase weight loss)							
GRAIN 1 ½ servings (limit or avoid to increase weight loss)							
RAW NUTS AND RAW SEEDS Limit to 1 to 2 handfuls							
FLAXSEED (fresh ground) 2 tablespoons							
AVOCADO ¼ to 1 small, 2 to 3 times per week							
MEAT OR FISH (optional) 3 to 4 ounces (limit to 4 times or fewer per week)							

USE THIS CHART AS A GUIDE

THE FIRST STEP

Eating an abundance of natural whole plant foods loaded with antioxidants gives us the ability to reclaim and maintain our health. After all, when antioxidant-rich foods are consumed, the body begins functioning more efficiently and replacing unhealthy cells with healthier ones.

Remember Genesis 1:29? "Behold, I give you every plant yielding seed that is on the surface of all the earth, and every tree which has fruit yielding seed; it shall be food for you . . ." Our Creator has always intended for us to eat whole plant foods.

As you begin eating this way, you will notice remarkable things happening to your body and mind. But optimal health is more than *eating* differently. You must also *think* and *act* differently.

• Adopt a warrior's attitude. Your desire to live life must outweigh the desire to give up. Don't choose to be the victim anymore!

• Make the determined decision to change. We all have the ability to change, and we don't have to do it alone.

• Forgive yourself. Learn to forgive yourself for bad choices, but be aware of what triggers them. Then practice avoiding those triggers.

• Discover new ways to embrace and enjoy life. Change is not easy. And when life's circumstances become difficult or a traumatic event happens, people sometimes give up. They find no joy in living, so they lose the will to live. I will share my experience.

Nine months after my accident and after religiously eating a high antioxidant diet, I was still suffering from excruciating IBS symptoms. I had tried many effective natural techniques, but my IBS symptoms always returned. The only relief I found was by not eating. I began losing weight.

One doctor said I looked too thin. I knew I needed to eat more, but I didn't want the IBS to return. I was so angry with my body that I felt betrayed. At that point, I decided to become even more fanatical in the pursuit of health. I persevered but each time I tried, I would experience another IBS attack.

Then I remembered that a couple of people had suggested I purchase Germaine Copeland's book *Prayers That Avail Much*, which contained scriptural prayers.

I went to the bookstore and glanced through the books on the shelf. At eye level, the only book lying against the back of the shelf with the cover facing me was the very book I needed: *Prayers That Avail Much.* I grabbed it, paid for it, raced out to my car, and began reading the healing prayers aloud while sitting in the driver's seat.

Later in my office, a sense of light filled the room. I realized that I had had the desire to be thin during my modeling days, but more memories erupted. I began thinking about my twin brother's death when we were eighteen. The loss had been too much for me to handle. I had thought I couldn't go on without him. During that time of loss, I subconsciously lost the will to live. I also realized the pattern of gorging and starving during my modeling days had been a way to comfort myself from the pain and loss. Then I realized that my health problems had left me feeling powerless,

forcing me to take stock of my life, my choices, and my situation.

I suddenly realized how blessed I was and how beautiful life could be. At that moment, I made a decision to love, embrace, and be grateful for my life. Instantly, the pain ceased. In less than two months, I felt healthier than ever before. My body's defenses became stronger and are still thriving today. The IBS episodes are now almost nonexistent.

In part 3 of this book, Journey to Wholeness, you will find exercises to assist you in your own self-discovery process. I also recommend a good life coach, counselor, or therapist to help guide you along the way. The first step, however, is to make the decision to adopt a warrior's attitude to live life and live it fully!

ANTI-INFLAMATION FOOD LIST

Vegetables
Bell peppers
Bok choy
Broccoli
Broccoli sprouts
Brussels sprouts
Cabbage
Cauliflower
Chard
Collards
Fennel bulb
Garlic
Green beans
Green onions
Kale
Leeks
Olives
Sea vegetables
Spinach
Sweet potatoes

Fruits
Acerola cherries
Apples
Avocados
Black currants
Blueberries
Fresh pineapple
Goji berries
Guavas
Kumquats
Lemons
Limes
Mulberries
Oranges
Papayas
Raspberries
Rhubarb
Strawberries
Tomatoes

Herbs and Spices
Basil
Cayenne pepper
Chili peppers
Cinnamon
Cocoa powder (natural)
Licorice
Mint
Oregano
Parsley
Rosemary
Thyme
Turmeric

Raw Nuts and Seeds
Almonds
Flaxseed
Hazelnuts
Sunflower seeds
Walnuts

Fish (wild, not farm-raised)
Anchovies
Herring
Mackerel
Rainbow trout
Salmon
Sardines

Drinks
Green tea
Herbal teas

PORTIONS CHART

Food	Amount	Portion
Bok choy, thinly sliced	1 cup	1 serving
Kale, destemmed and chopped	1 cup	1 serving
Broccoli florets	1½ cups	1 serving
Celery	2 stalks	1 serving
Carrot	1 medium	1 serving
Romaine lettuce	2 cups	1 serving
Cauliflower florets	4 medium	1 serving
Zucchini	1 large	1 serving
Cooked legumes	1 cup	1 serving
Cabbage, shredded	1 cup	1 serving
Bell pepper, seeded	1 large	3 servings
Roma tomato	1 medium	1 serving
Romaine and mixed raw chopped/shredded vegetable salad	2 heaping cups	1 serving
Fruits	1 hand sized fruit	1 serving
Berries	1 cup	1 serving
Cut-up fruit	½ cup	1 serving

CHAPTER THREE

THE PATH TO OPTIMAL HEALTH

LOSING WEIGHT

My goal for writing this book is to provide the tools for achieving overall optimal health. One by-product of optimal health is ideal weight. Although most people achieve their ideal weight by following the Super Antioxidant Diet, some people have difficulty during the early phases.

Studies indicate that each person has a set-point weight, a weight the body interprets as ideal. Sometimes, if we've been overweight for some time, we have to retrain our bodies to get used to less weight.

Body weight tends to be regulated, and the hypothalamus gland makes sure of that! It monitors body fat content and tells us when we are hungry or full. If our body weight gets below a certain point, a whole set of signals is produced to influence the need for food. Without food, the metabolism, or basal metabolic rate (BMR), slows down. The body interprets this lack of food as a starvation threat and it slows down to save energy. It also takes less energy for a lighter person to move around.

For some overweight individuals, the presence of excess fat may compound the problem. When the body acquires extra fat cells, these cells apparently fight to stay the same size. This may prompt you to eat more.

The set-point theory may explain why gaining and losing weight can be equally difficult and why some people get stuck on plateaus. To minimize the possibility of this happening, you should:

• Lose weight slowly. Crash dieting can permanently lower your BMR and even cause you to gain weight on few calories.

Losing one to one and a half pounds of fat a week is an excellent goal. If done gradually, you will reset your set-point weight.

• Avoid late-night eating. Some individuals wake up during the night to eat. If you cannot break this habit, I suggest you get some counseling. I also recommend a consultation with a sleep specialist.

• Be aware of how much you are eating. People automatically crave excess fat and calories in order to maintain individual set points. Even on the Super Antioxidant Diet, people who are eating correctly fail to note the exact amount of nuts and other fatty foods they are consuming.

• Get regular exercise. Consistent exercise increases metabolic function.

OVERCOMING OBSTACLES

Most people have not had the opportunity to experience optimal health even though they know all about healthy eating. Why? These seven obstacles can keep us from achieving optimal health.

Confusion • Doubt • Food Cravings • Digestive Disturbances • Detoxification

Comfort • Peer Pressure

CONFUSION

There are so many diet plans bombarding us today, and few of them are based on facts. How do we know what to believe?

The Super Antioxidant Diet is based on dietary principals that have been validated by peer-reviewed, published scientific research. I have tried, however, not to burden you with too much technical information. (If you would like to learn more, you can find recommended reading in the resources section at the back of the book.) Nonetheless, you do need to know a few facts about your new eating plan so you won't be confused.

DAILY PROTEIN REQUIREMENTS

Dr. Couey writes in his university textbook *Nutrition for God's Temple*[1] that the recommended daily allowances (RDA) for protein is a guideline and varies with both weight and age. Infants, because of their tremendous rate of growth, need more than double that, or 2.2 grams per kilogram of body weight. The need gradually decreases with age until adulthood is reached. Of course, this is not dependent on age but on growth requirements. In addition, the RDA allots extra grams of protein during pregnancy (plus thirty grams) and while lactating (plus twenty grams).

The government RDA recommends fifty-six grams of protein for an average male and forty-four grams for an average female, this calculation being based on the reference male weighing 154 pounds (70 kilograms) and the reference female weighing 121 pounds (55 kilograms). Protein needs vary from individual to individual depending on several factors such as energy output and body size, so the RDA is very generous in its recommendations.

Notice, the RDA is a *recommended* amount, not a *required* amount. Recent studies reveal that consuming more than the RDA of animal protein has proven to be dangerous to our health. And what about all those high animal-protein diets?

American nutritional biochemistry scientist T. Colin Campbell, PhD, has been at the forefront of nutritional research, the results of which he reports in his book *The China Study.* The *New York Times* stated that Campbell's work is the most comprehensive study of the relationship between diet and the risk of developing disease. According to Dr. Campbell, "People who ate the most plant-based foods were the health and tended to avoid chronic disease."[2]

The Super Antioxidant Diet recipes in this book provide you with a daily protein intake above the required minimum, but keep animal protein to a minimum. A variety of high antioxidant plant foods provide ample protein as well as disease protection. A variety of vegetables, beans, nuts, and seeds throughout the day will provide you with all the necessary proteins. If you doubt me, read this ancient passage from the Bible:

Please test your servants for ten days, and let us be given some vegetables to eat and water to drink. Then let our appearance be observed in your presence and the appearance of the youths who are eating the king's choice food; and deal with your servants according to what you see. So he listened to them in this matter and tested them for ten days. At the end of ten days their appearance seemed better and they were fatter than all the youths who had been eating the king's choice food. So the overseer continued to withhold their choice food and the wine they were to drink, and kept giving them vegetables. As for these four youths, God gave them knowledge and intelligence in every branch of literature and wisdom; Daniel even understood all kinds of visions and dreams (Daniel 1:12–17).

COMBINING FOOD TYPES

Many people are misinformed about combining food types. They believe they must always combine certain plant foods to obtain necessary essential amino acids. The book *Diet for a Small Planet,* which emphasized the need for combining grains and beans at one meal, popularized this idea.[3] The author, Frances Moore Lappé, was being overly cautious in order to avoid criticism from the "nutrition establishment." Lappé later explained, "In combating the myth that meat is the only way to get high-quality protein, I reinforced another myth."[4]

DOUBT

Doubting in our ability to accomplish a goal can keep us from achieving it. The goal may be to lose weight, find a new job, get out of a bad relationship, or make some other change. But when we go against what we are used to doing, we have a tendency to hesitate. After all,

changing means we may need to go outside our comfort zone.

Have you noticed when you try to tell someone about something helpful that requires change, they often look at you with a glassy stare? Then they attempt to change the subject or make excuses. If you talk long enough, they may even get defensive and hostile. It doesn't matter if the information is true. It is still perceived as a threat.

Many of us try to talk ourselves out of hearing the truth by avoiding it. We ignore it or get too busy to think about it. We make excuses. And then we get upset at ourselves for ignoring it. Even when we *want* to change, old patterns kick in.

We learn patterns of coping at an early age. We are simply programmed not only to doubt our goals, based on past failures, but also to *fear subconsciously* what might happen if we actually *do* reach our goals. This doubt may not only influence behavior, but also influence brain chemistry.

Bruce Lipton, PhD, a cellular biologist, is an internationally recognized authority on bridging science and spirit. In his book *The Biology of Belief,* he relates a dramatic true story as told in the film *Shine* to illustrate the power of the subconscious mind:

In the movie . . . Australian concert pianist David Helfgott defies his father by going off to London to study music. Helfgott's father, a survivor of the Holocaust, programmed his son's subconscious mind with the belief that the world was unsafe, that if he "stood out" it might be life threatening. His father insisted he would be safe only if he stayed close to his family. In spite of his father's relentless programming, Helfgott knew that he was a world-class pianist who needed to break from his father to realize his dream.[5]

While Helfgott plays a notoriously difficult piano piece, the film depicts the conflict between his conscious mind *wanting success* and his subconscious mind *fearing that success.* He labors to play to the end, and manages to do so. After the last note, he passes out, overcome by the exhaustion of battling his fears.

Dr. Lipton writes, "Most of us engage in less dramatic battles with our subconscious mind as we try to undo the programming we received as children. Witness our ability to continually seek out jobs that we fail at, or remain in jobs we hate, because we don't 'deserve' a better life."

FOOD CRAVINGS

Food cravings are the body's cry for nutrients. Sensitive sensors in the digestive tract signal the hypothalamus to turn off the hunger drive when one has consumed the necessary fat, protein, fiber, calories, vitamins, and minerals.[6] Until one consumes enough of these necessary nutrients, the hypothalamus gland will continue to signal one to keep eating.

In today's culture, people consume too much fat, protein, and calories and lack the nutrients that plant foods provide. A hamburger or piece of cheesy lasagna or fried chicken may satisfy one's caloric and fat needs, but hunger will return because important nutritional needs including antioxidants have not been satisfied.

The recipes and meal plans in the Super Antioxidant Diet have been designed to supply all nutritional needs, thus triggering the turn-off switch to this physiological hunger drive.

DIGESTIVE DISTURBANCES

Because antioxidant rich foods contain fiber, you may experience some digestive disturbances while on the Super Antioxidant Diet. The good news is that you can recalibrate your digestive tract to efficiently process a nutrient-rich diet, but it takes some time and patience. The benefits are well worth it.

If you suffer from any chronic colon condition, such as IBS, colitis, or diverticulitis, talk with your medical doctor before beginning this diet. I recommend that you work with a nutritionist or a nutritionally knowledgeable medical doctor to help you.

DETOXIFICATION

Eating a lot of meat, processed foods, starchy foods, and sugar interferes with the body's ability to cleanse itself of toxins and cellular trash. When you eliminate unhealthy foods and begin consuming more antioxidant rich foods, your body begins the process of detoxifying and repairing.

Usually, during the first few days on the Super Antioxidant Diet, you will feel great, but eventually you will encounter the lurking dragon: your addiction to unhealthy food. You may experience hunger pangs, body aches, headaches, and tiredness. *Don't give up. The phase doesn't last too long.*

Detoxification involves more than just the physical body. Our beings include the body (physical), soul (mind and emotions), and spirit (life force). When one aspect begins to detoxify, another will follow. *We must be willing to go through the uncomfortable detoxification process to stay on the plan.*

When I began eating this way, I had to take charge of my thought life. My body was working hard to repair while my thoughts were busy telling me I didn't have the strength to get through it. I had to learn the facts to fight my dragon of fear. My body did heal itself. I have detoxified greatly and continue to do so.

The Super Antioxidant Diet causes detoxification to begin with the physical aspect but allows detoxification to take place in all areas of your life.

COMFORT

Our brains are designed to reward with good feelings by releasing natural pleasure chemicals when we do what we are designed to do. When we become hungry and do not satisfy our hunger, we experience discomfort. We are therefore motivated to eat to avoid this discomfort.

The Pleasure Trap, by Douglas J. Lisle, PhD, and Alan Goldhamer, DC, explains in detail how we are motivated by a primal motivation triad: seeking pleasure, avoidance of pain, and conservation of energy.[7] *The Pleasure Trap* explains how cravings work and how to overcome them.

Primitive man's foraged food was rich in antioxidant nutrients and fiber but low in calories—the ideal diet. He had a difficult time foraging enough food to get the required calories to sustain and reproduce life. He was rewarded with pleasure chemicals for motivation to consume enough food for survival.

Unlike primitive man, today we are surrounded by high-calorie foods that release pleasure chemicals, quickly satisfy our hunger, and take very little energy to obtain. High-calorie foods provide the quick unhealthy fix that keeps a person addicted.

The more stress in your life, the more pleasure chemicals you want. The more calories you consume, the more feel-good brain chemicals you receive. It becomes an endless cycle.

Inappropriately stimulated brain chemicals can be powerful drugs, and it takes some time to withdraw. For this reason, I suggest getting regular counseling or coaching, immersing yourself in factual health information, avoiding nonsupportive people, spending time with supportive people, and consciously working on reprogramming your brain.

PEER PRESSURE

You can't go anywhere without encountering peer pressure. There's peer pressure in the media, in the workplace, in the family, at church, at social gatherings, amongst friends and even strangers. It will never go away, so we just have to find a healthy way to cope with it.

Being aware is the first step. We can make peer pressure work for us by creating a core group of supportive peers with whom to connect. Often we go along with the crowd because we don't want to look foolish or seem unsocial. And quite frankly, much of our social life revolves around eating. We go to dinner parties, weddings, holiday parties, restaurants with friends, and church and temple socials where donuts and coffee are served.

Peer pressure is an extremely powerful motivator because it stems from a primal need. Early humans had to band together in groups or tribes because there was safety in numbers. Outside the tribe there were many dangers—marauding tribes and wild animals—that could overcome a single person. Being rejected by our peer group triggers a deep-rooted primal fear of not being able to survive.

It is important to find or create social outlets to share this lifestyle with others. Get a group of people together to have healthy dinner clubs where you can try different antioxidant dishes, support each other, and discuss how to live more healthfully. The most effective way to utilize this diet/lifestyle is to be motivated by rewards rather than the feeling of fear and deprivation.

CHAPTER FOUR

SYSTEM RECALIBRATION

Whenever our dietary pattern changes, our bodies must recalibrate hormone production, brain-chemical production, digestive juices, blood flow, and so on. The body is designed to maintain a stable, constant chemical condition called "homeostasis." This state motivates us to maintain the norm: the same amount of calories, fat, protein, sugar, caffeine, alcohol, and other drugs.

When we change our eating habits, we upset the balance and our bodies must recalibrate. It's during this time that we are *most vulnerable.* We will encounter unpleasant symptoms and mind games.

Don't be fooled. There are many quick-fix remedies on the market today just waiting to grab your money. You may have already tried them.

The key is time. Time is what you need to detoxify your cells. Time is what your body needs to replace unhealthy cells with healthier ones. Time will help you successfully recalibrate a mindset, an

unhealthy eating pattern, and a negative way of coping.

Think of your body as a house with a good foundation. It's just that the structure has begun to fall apart. In order to rebuild your house in a healthy way, you need to deconstruct, or get rid of, all those weak materials. This process can be somewhat unpleasant.

To begin your body's deconstruction process, your must first eliminate your consumption of and exposure to toxic materials. This is necessary to allow your body to purge itself of unhealthy cells and toxins. Following the Super Antioxidant Diet will ensure that your body does this gently and naturally at just the right pace for you.

As mentioned previously in the book, you may experience hunger pangs, headaches, body aches, and tiredness. You may also experience gas pains because of diet change. Be kind to yourself during this time. If you choose to return to old eating patterns or use stimulants, you will prolong the deconstruction process. Have patience. The building has only begun.

RECONSTRUCTION

The process of reconstruction begins with change. With the Super Antioxidant Diet, you will begin noticing small changes: weight loss, glowing skin, increased bowel movements, and a more positive attitude.

You are now rebuilding your home with the highest quality materials. If you follow the Super Antioxidant Diet and continue increasing your antioxidant intake, you will start experiencing a greater sense of well-being and energy. Your body has begun reconstructing, and the detoxification process will become intermittent. You will become more familiar and comfortable with your body's detoxification signals.

The basic construction of your healthy new home is now complete.

ENHANCED CONSTRUCTION

By increasing your antioxidant rich vegetable and fruit intake, especially raw foods, you leave less room for animal products and unhealthy, processed foods.

And because raw foods contain live enzymes that aid in digestion, adding more of them will help you feel refreshed and rejuvenated.

You should consult your doctor, of course, if you have any medical concern that may prevent you from adding more raw vegetables to your diet.

During the Enhanced Construction phase, you may experience:

• Healthy weight

• Smoother, more elastic skin

• Abundant energy

• Mental clarity

• Increased stamina

• Glowing skin

• A growing desire for healthy foods

CHAPTER FIVE

THE SEVENFOLD PLAN

The number seven in Hebrew numerology or *Gematria* is interpreted as being the "perfect" or "complete" number. Make the commitment to follow the Super Antioxidant Diet for seven weeks. See if you don't experience positive changes. The sevenfold plan includes:

- Diet

- Water

- Physical exercise

- Rest

- Awareness

- Fresh air and sunshine

- Personal hygiene

Diet: Every seven days make a new commitment to follow the plan for another seven days.

Water: By following the Super Antioxidant Diet, you will get water in its purest form from the food you eat. When you get thirsty or need water for food preparation, I recommend water with a pH of 7.2 or higher. Fiji brand water has a pH of 7.5.

Physical Exercise: Follow our Move Your Body moderate exercise plan or a more rigorous program after consulting your doctor. I try to get some form of exercise seven days a week.

Rest: Try to get a good night's sleep, at least seven (optimally, eight) hours of sleep each night. Medical evidence recommends the average adult should get seven to nine hours of sleep daily.[1] In most cases, insomnia appears to be caused by too much activity and worry.

In Western societies, chronic sleep disorders are common. Sleep disorders can be symptoms of certain physical and psychological illnesses such as heart and lung problems, acid reflux, allergies, arthritis, cancer, fibromyalgia, prostate problems, hormone imbalance, Alzheimer's disease, Parkinson's disease, hyperthyroidism, sleep apnea, restless leg syndrome, and leg cramps. If you suffer from insomnia, I recommend you see your physician to determine if there is an underlying cause.

The health consequences of sleep deprivation put us at risk for weight gain, diabetes, heart disease, stroke, and memory loss.

Many people suffer from lack of restorative sleep. They work excessively to make ends meet and fail to go to sleep when they are tired. People drink caffeinated beverages to keep going when they should be pausing for some rest. The body requests sleep in two ways: by increasing the levels of a certain neurotransmitter and by the body's circadian clock. The sleep neurotransmitter acts as a slow-down switch, signaling the body to feel tired and drowsy. Caffeine blocks the neurotransmitter and the clue to rest is missed.

Sleep is vitally important for health. Laboratory rats deprived of sleep for more than a week suffered severe loss of immune function. Human studies have shown that participants who slept only fours hours for six consecutive days developed higher blood pressure and higher stress hormone (cortisol) levels, considerably reduced number of antibodies, insulin resistance, impaired

memory and reaction time, and metabolic slowdown. All of these symptoms were reversed when the participants made up the missed hours of sleep.[2] Recent evidence indicates that sleep deprivation may increase the risk of cancer, diabetes, obesity, emotional and psychological problems, and even death.

In the United States, the market for pharmaceutical sleep aids is at an all-time high. These drugs can cause a host of problems including dependence.[3] In our modern world, we have distanced ourselves so far from our Creator's instructions. I understand why the Sabbath rest was emphasized so many times in the Bible. We simply were not designed to work seven days per week. Studies not only support Biblical dietary laws but also affirm the need for rest. Personally, I made the decision to rest on Saturday, the Biblical Sabbath, the seventh day of the week. I have experienced numerous benefits from this decision.

By going nonstop, we throw our systems way out of whack, and then wonder why we are suffering from insomnia and a host of other related ailments. Prescription pill popping may temporarily help while we get back on track, but not for long.

Here are some tips for getting a good night's sleep:

• Don't eat for at least three hours before going to sleep. And eat for nutrition's sake, not for other reasons such as entertainment. Eating while performing other tasks can form associations that are difficult to break. For instance, eating while in bed or watching television can associate food with relaxation.

• Get some type of daily exercise. Even a little exercise can help you relax at the end of the day, but try not to exercise close to bedtime.

• Try wearing an eye mask. Darkness stimulates your brain to produce sleep chemicals. We are not designed to sleep in artificial light.

• Try earplugs. We are not designed to sleep through urban noise.

• Go to sleep around the same time every night.

• Develop calming bedtime rituals such as reading something enjoyable or taking a bath.

• Do not watch disturbing television shows before retiring.

• Avoid stimulating conversations or creative projects before retiring.

• If you find yourself awake in the middle of the night, think of pleasant things, pray for yourself and others, go over your numerous blessings, and be grateful for these quiet moments to develop an attitude of gratitude. By lying still and filling yourself with pleasant thoughts, you will find yourself feeling rested the following day.

• I recommend Transformation CalmZyme supplement, which is uniquely formulated with natural enzymes and nutrients to assist the body with stress relief and to enhance the quality of sleep.

Reset your circadian rhythm by going out in the daylight for at least ten minutes immediately upon rising in the morning—that is, if you arise during morning daylight hours. Circadian refers to a daily cycle. The circadian rhythm is commonly referred to as the biological clock. It is the rhythm of sleep and wakefulness.

Awareness: The Journey to Wholeness exercises in this book are designed to help you become aware of what you need to find balance and moderation in your life. The more aware you become, the more easily you will find the strength to move away from self-destructive behaviors.

I suggest setting aside a certain time of day to read words of reinforcement and wisdom. My favorites are the Proverbs. They are generic yet practical and meaningful.

Fresh Air and Sunshine: To get the vitamin D you need for healthy bones, you need to be in the sun for fifteen minutes per day. Just be careful not to get excessive sun, as it can be damaging.[4,5]

Personal Hygiene: Our overall health is impacted by what we eat and what we come in contact with. And because the Super Antioxidant Diet is about holistic health, I recommend you use natural body-care products.

You should also floss your teeth regularly. The American Academy of Periodontology has linked periodontal (gum) disease to heart disease.[6]

These natural products can be found in health food stores and in the health care sections of most supermarkets:

Toothpaste • Mouthwash
Soap • Facial cleanser
Moisturizer • Lotion
Cosmetics • Bath products
Hair products • Hair
coloring products

CHAPTER SIX

BARE MINIMUM SUPPLEMENTS

Supplements are meant to supplement, not replace. Because the Super Antioxidant Diet is nutrient packed, you will require only a few supplements to support your new dietary style.

Initially, researchers thought that consuming certain nutrients in pill form would be adequate but not so. Researchers still haven't even been able to identify many of the nutrients found in food, much less package them. They now conclude that the most promising research in preventing disease relates to dietary habits, not nutritional supplements.

I recommend only food-based, nonsynthetic supplements. These include:

Vitamin D • Calcium • Essential
fatty acids • Probiotics
Enzymes • Vitamin B-12
Iron • Pomegranate

VITAMIN D

You cannot get sufficient vitamin D from food. The problem seems to be that we are not getting enough vitamin D with sun exposure either. Since we all know that too much exposure to the sun is damaging, many doctors recommend a supplement of vitamin D.

The Institute of Medicine determined insufficient scientific information to establish an RDA for vitamin D. Instead, they established the measurement of adequate intake (AI), which represents a daily vitamin D intake to maintain bone health and normal calcium metabolism in most healthy people. Vitamin D is the most toxic of all vitamins. Never exceed more than two and a half times the AI.[1]

AGE	VITAMIN D AI
14–18 years	200 IU
19–50 years	200 IU
51–70 years	400 IU
71 years plus	600 IU

CALCIUM

The RDA for calcium is between 1,000 to 1,300 mg for both men and women, depending on age. Dr. Fuhrman's Osteo-Sun is an excellent choice. But remember, even the best diet and calcium supplements won't properly benefit you without the inclusion of weight-bearing exercises.

ESSENTIAL FATTY ACIDS

DHA (docosahexaenoic acid) is an omega-3 fat that helps prevent inflammation and is important for brain function. DHA is also produced in small amounts from the body's enzymatic conversion of other omega-3 fatty acids (such as a-linolenic acid, or ALA) found in certain foods. The foods rich in omega-3 fats are flaxseed, walnuts, soybeans, and other seeds and nuts.

Fish oil is high in the already converted DHA. Most of the DHA in fish and other more complex organisms originates in microalgae and collects in greater quantities in prey organisms as they move up the food chain.

Low levels of DHA cause reduction of important brain chemicals and has been associated with ADHD (attention deficit/hyperactivity disorder), Alzheimer's disease, and depression. There is growing evidence that DHA supplementation may be effective in combating such diseases.

If you have inflammatory disorders, Transformation's EFA (essential fatty acid) supplementation is recommended. Dr. Fuhrman's DHA Purity, derived from microalgae, is an excellent brand for vegans.

PROBIOTICS

Probiotics are live microorganisms that benefit the digestive tract by improving the balance of the intestinal bacterial flora.

For proper digestion to take place, food must be broken down into a form that allows nutrients to be absorbed by our bodies. To do so, our cells produce enzymes that break down the food into smaller and smaller particles that are passed through the cells' membranes into the cells.

Alone, these enzymes are insufficient. Colonies of friendly bacteria in the intestine are necessary to complete the digestive process. By supplementing with friendly bacteria (probiotics), we increase the capacity to digest food and absorb nutrients.

The role of friendly intestinal bacterial flora is to occupy the intestinal tract, thus preventing the unfriendly bacteria from becoming predominant. If the latter occurs, inflammation of the bowels and other disorders arise. When we take antibiotics to fight an infection, for instance, we may experience diarrhea. Antibiotics kill friendly bacteria, which leaves the intestinal tract vulnerable to the overgrowth of unfriendly bacteria. A quality probiotic supplement reintroduces the friendly bacteria into our digestive systems. The friendly bacteria help create a barrier on the intestinal wall that stops the unfriendly bacteria from invading cells.

The use of live microorganisms for health has a long history. It is mentioned in the Bible and other sacred books in the form of cultured dairy products and cultured vegetables.

Today, probiotics come in liquid, powder, or pills. We recommend Transformation Enzymes' Plantadophilus or TPP Probiotic (see transformationenzymes.com). I also recommend Bio-K Plus, the powerful probiotic that has done wonders for me and other people with colon disorders. This product is quite expensive but has shown promising results with numerous intestinal disorders. To learn more about Bio-K Plus, visit biokplus.com

ENZYMES

We know the importance of proper nutrition to health and wellness, but nutrition is not limited to healthy foods or high-quality supplements. We must also digest, transport, and absorb those essential nutrients and then eliminate the by-products.

A digestive system that fails to process food for availability and absorption will undermine the body's coping ability and create conditions favorable for disease and metabolic disorders. Additionally, genetics, lifestyle, stress, and the environment impact our digestive function on a daily basis. Digestive enzymes help the overtaxed body to digest and absorb nutrients.

There are many supplement companies that produce enzyme supplements. Because it is difficult to know what companies produce quality supplements, we recommend Transformation Enzyme Corporation's (TEC) digestive enzymes (see transformationenzymes.com). TEC researches and formulates an extensive line of pharmaceutical-grade digestive enzyme supplements designed exclusively for licensed or certified health care professionals. TEC is considered one of the pioneer companies in the field of supplemental digestive enzymes with more than twenty years of experience.

The following supplements are recommend if you are eating the Super Antioxidant Diet and want to:

Speed up your recovery time:

• Transformation's DigestZyme or TPP Digest. These formulas provide support to the pancreas and gallbladder, two organs that tend to be overburdened by the Standard American Diet. These digestive formulas reduce food intolerances, promote nutrient bioavailability, reduce oxidative stress, and promote a strong immune system.

• Transformation's PureZyme or TPP Protease. These proteolytic formulas improve circulation, modulate immune function, increase resistance to infections, reduce inflammation, and support the body's detoxification systems.

• Transformation's Plantadophilus or TPP Probiotic.

Reverse and prevent inflammation disorders:

• Transformation's Essential Fatty Acids (EFA) is manufactured from a highly purified fish oil concentrate and is a rich source of omega-3 fatty acids. A diet rich in essential fatty acids can promote cardiovascular health as well as help control and reduce inflammation.

• Transformation's TPP Protease IFC is a blend of proteases, bromelain, papain, and antioxidants specifically formulated for their anti-inflammatory properties. This product is ideal for reducing inflammatory conditions associated with allergies, arthritis, cardiovascular disease, or tissue damage resulting from injuries, sports workouts, or even surgical procedures.

The following are other helpful supplements:

• Transformation's Super CellZyme, a whole-food vitamin and mineral supplement formulated with enzymes to facilitate the absorption of these nutrients into the cell.

• Transformation's CalmZyme, an herbal/enzyme formula designed to help your body and nervous system relax. It is an excellent support for insomnia, hypertension, headaches, anxiety, and hyperactivity, and may assist with neurotransmitter regulation to help mood disorders.

VITAMIN B-12

Vitamin B-12's primary functions are in the formation of red blood cells and the maintenance of a healthy nervous system. B-12 is necessary for the rapid synthesis of DNA during cell division. Bacteria that are found primarily in meat, eggs, and dairy products produce B-12.

When B-12 deficiency occurs, DNA production is disrupted. Symptoms of B-12 deficiency include excessive tiredness, breathlessness, listlessness, pallor, and poor resistance to infection. Other symptoms can include a smooth, sore tongue and menstrual disorders. Vitamin B-12 neuropathy, involving the degeneration of nerve fibers and irreversible neurological damage, can also occur.

As we get older, it becomes more difficult to absorb vitamin B-12. It is also tough for vegans (vegetarians who only eat only plant foods) to get enough B-12. If you are a vegetarian and especially a vegan, B-12 supplementation is strongly advised.

A sublingual B-12 is a relatively inexpensive supplement that can be purchased at any health food store or in the natural vitamin section of most supermarkets. Follow the dosage instructions on the label. You can also get B-12 injections from your physician.

IRON

If you are following a vegan diet, you may need to supplement with iron. On the Super Antioxidant Diet, you will eat plenty of dark green leafy vegetables that supply adequate amounts of iron. You should only take iron if your doctor determines you need it.

POMEGRANATE

Overwhelming evidence demonstrates the health benefits of the antioxidants found in pomegranate fruit.[2,3,4] Life Extension has added standardized pomegranate extract to its supplement line (you can order Life Extension Pomegranate Extract Capsules at lef.org or by calling 800-544-4440). Consult with your physician before using this product if you are taking anti-seizure, antidepressant, or psychiatric medications, certain types of blood pressure medications (e.g., calcium channel blockers), or cholesterol reduction medications (e.g., statins).

For more information on supplements, visit www.vibrantcuisine.com.

PART II

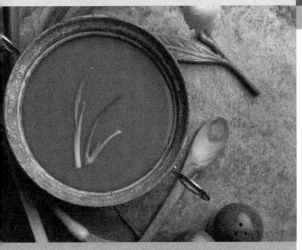

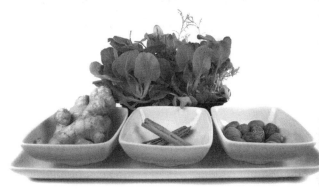

VIBRANT CUISINE

*Never put off until tommorow
what you can do today.*

One of my former employers gave me the initial inspiration for writing this book. He taught me to pursue my dreams in a focused, practical manner. Part of the advice I got from him was: *Do It Now!* I try to do everything in the *now,* instead of putting it off.

Since I have been writing this book, I have encountered frustrating obstacles. Thankfully, I have overcome these challenges with the help of my Creator, friends, and family. I have seen other people give in to *giving up,* and it's usually when they are on the verge of accomplishing something important. When we persevere, we become stronger and even more determined.

I'm a fellow traveler on this journey. For instance, I was suffering from esophageal pain (damage from my horseback-riding accident) and I needed to complete the final work on the book. I also had a lot to do to prepare for another six-week teaching session. I was being tempted to listen to that internal "victim" dialogue, which made me feel even more insecure. How could I teach people to achieve good health if I didn't feel well myself?

That day I had an appointment with my life coach. During our meeting, I realized what I had already known subconsciously: I am only a *messenger* of health and I am on the same journey. It's my responsibility to pass along the knowledge that has been given to me.

If you face similar challenges, remember: *There is no time like now!*

CHAPTER SEVEN

TAKE ACTION

In this section, I share with you the recipes I have created over the past twenty years. Eventually, you should build on what I have learned and create your own Vibrant Cuisine recipes. Until then, use the meal guides for the menu plan of your preference.

This book provides three weeks of daily meal guides for these four plans:

- Meat and Fish Eaters Plan

- Fish Eaters Plan

- Ultimate Vegan Plan

- Anti-Inflammation Plan

Many recipes make large portions and people have plenty of leftovers for the week. Portions can be frozen as well. Prep plenty of salad, too. It will last you all week!

Here are some hints to help you maximize your antioxidant recipes.

SEASONINGS

Salt: Most of my recipes are prepared with little or no salt because salt consumption has been linked to both stomach cancer and high blood pressure.[1] Salt also causes our taste buds to become desensitized to natural taste and flavors. In addition, salt causes calcium and other trace minerals to be leached from the body, which contributes to osteoporosis.[2]

The RDA for sodium is only 500 mg, so keep your sodium intake at 500 mg or less. If you eat an antioxidant diet loaded with vegetables, you will naturally get around 300 mg of sodium. I recommend very small amounts of Bragg Liquid Amino Acids or unrefined sea salt, which can be found at most health food stores or in the natural products section of many supermarkets.

One-half teaspoon of table or sea salt contains about 1,200 mg of sodium whereas one-half teaspoon of Bragg Liquid Amino Acids contains only 120 mg. Bragg Liquid Amino Acids tastes similar to soy sauce.[3] It even comes in a spray bottle, so you can spray it on the surface of the food after serving. It has a nice robust flavor that many people find enhances foods.

If you are a heavy salt eater, you will probably experience some salt withdrawal. It can take a couple of months to regain your natural taste sensitivity.

Black Pepper: I do not use black pepper in my recipes. Black pepper can be irritating to digestive tracts, especially those with acid reflux or ulcers. Also, highly spiced foods have been linked to esophageal cancer.[4,5]

Natural Spices and Herbs: Most of my recipes are moderately seasoned. My goal is for you to be creative with seasoning these recipes to your taste, so add preferred natural spices and herbs.

FATS

Cooking Oil: I limit the use of oil in cooking because we should receive plenty of fat from whole foods (avocados, nuts, and seeds). If you choose to use oil, use a very small amount of cold-pressed olive oil, nut oil, or seed oil. Do not heat the oil because heating changes the molecular structure. Instead, just drizzle it on after the food is cooked.

Natural Fats: If you are trying to gain weight or are athletically active, you may wish to eat more avocados, an extra handful of nuts, more beans, additional starchy vegetables and grains, and a little additional oil if you like. Be sure you don't fill up on these items but continue to consume antioxidant-rich leafy greens, green and colored vegetables, and fruits.

CHAPTER EIGHT

KITCHEN MAKEOVER

Get rid of junk food (sweets, processed foods, salty foods, and *anything else* that is unhealthy) from your home. If family members do not share your desire to eat healthfully, create separate areas of the kitchen for yourself that include:

- Helpful appliances and utensils

- Pantry of whole foods and salt-free seasonings

- Refrigerator/freezer of whole foods

HELPFUL APPLIANCES AND UTENSILS

It's a good idea to purchase these items, if you don't have them already:

Baking pans
Blender
Chinese wok
Citrus juice squeezer
Clay pot for baking (Romertopf is a good brand)
Colander
Cookware (stainless steel or enamel)
Crock pot
Food containers (for leftovers)
Food processor
Food scale (an inexpensive one is all you need)
Garlic press
Grater
Hand mixer
Hot pad holders

Electric ice cream maker
Juicer (Jack LaLanne has an
inexpensive, excellent brand)

Knives:
Chef's knife
Paring knives

Measuring cups
Micro plane (fine grater)
Mixing bowls (set)
Pressure cooker
Pyrex baking dishes
Salad spinner
Spatulas (rubber)

Spoons:
Wooden spoons
Large cooking spoon
Measuring spoons
Slotted spoon

Soup kettle (large)
Strainer
Timer
Vegetable peeler
Wire whisk

FILLING THE PANTRY

General:
Arrowroot or corn starch
Baking powder
Baking soda
Miso (white miso has the least
sodium)
Nutritional yeast (available in
health food stores)
100% fruit spread
Sea vegetables (arame, hizki,
kombu, mekabu, wakame)

Oils:
Olive oil (cold-pressed, virgin)
Olive oil (spray)
Sesame oil (toasted)

Spices and Seasonings:
Caraway seeds
Chili powders
Cinnamon
Crushed red pepper
Curry powder
Garam masala (available in
health food or Indian stores)
Garlic powder
Herbs (dried, any variety)
No-salt herb seasonings
Onions (dried)
Sweet Hungarian paprika

Smoked paprika
Turmeric
Unrefined sea salt (use
extremely sparingly—½ tsp
contains 1200 mg sodium)
Vanilla extract

Dried Fruits (sulfite-free):
Blueberries (unsweetened)
Cherries (unsweetened)
Currants
Dates
Goji berries
Mango (unsweetened)
Raisins (avoid white raisins
because they contain sulfites)

Soups, Bouillons, and Broths:
Chicken broth (salt-free)
No-salt or low-salt soup base
seasoning
Rapunzel Salt-Free Bouillon
cubes (health food store—use
sparingly, high in fat)
Vegetable broth (salt-free)

Seasoned Liquids and Sauces:
Balsamic vinegar
Bragg Liquid Amino Acids

Ketchup (natural)
Pasta sauce (low sodium)
Salad dressings (preservative-
free and fat-free or low-fat nat-
ural and the lowest sodium)
Seasoned vinegars
Tabasco
Worcestershire sauce

Sweeteners:
Date sugar (from health food store)
Honey (use very sparingly)
Maple syrup (use very sparingly)
Stevia (use very sparingly)
Xylitol (use very sparingly)

Canned Goods:
All types of canned salt-free
beans and legumes
Aseptic carton natural soups
Green chilies
Natural bean and vegetable
soups (preferably salt-free)
Tomatoes (whole or crushed
without excess sodium)
Tomato paste (without
excess sodium)
Tomato puree (without
excess sodium)

Dried Beans or Legumes:
Adzuki beans
Anastazi beans
Black beans
Butter or lima beans
Canellini beans
Fava beans
French flageolet beans
Garbanzo beans
Great Northern beans
Lentils (green, French, black, red)
Navy beans
Pinto beans
Soybeans
Split peas (green and yellow)

Drinks:
Herbal or green tea
Pomegranate juice (unsweetened)
Soy milk
Veggie juice (no or low sodium)

Nuts and Seeds:
Almonds
Cashews
Macadamias
Natural peanut butter (sugar-free, salt-free)
Pistachios
Poppy seeds
Pumpkin seeds
Raw nut butters

Sesame seeds (unhulled)
Sunflower seeds
Tahini (sesame seed paste)
Walnuts
Whole flaxseed

Whole Grains:
Basmati brown rice
Bhutanese red rice
Chinese black rice
Jasmine brown rice
Long grain brown rice
Oatmeal
Polenta
Quinoa
Short grain brown rice
Wehani rice
Wheat berries
Whole barley
Wild rice

STOCKING THE FREEZER

Feel free to use frozen vegetables as often as you like. Remember, they are almost as nutrient dense as fresh vegetables and sometimes even more so. Frozen combinations, such as Asian or Southwestern, work fine as well. Make sure to read the labels to *avoid any that contain chemical additives or excessive salt.*

CHAPTER NINE

EXPRESS SHOPPING

Shopping twice a week should be sufficient. Shop more if you like. The produce section of the supermarket is where you will spend most of your time, so stay away from the processed food aisles. Even so, products labeled "natural" may still contain chemical additives. Better yet, organic food co-ops and farmers' markets will provide you with the freshest produce possible.

Make sure to purchase seasonal fruits and vegetables, as they are always the most nutrient dense. Fruits and vegetables are often waxed to retain moisture content. If possible, purchase unwaxed produce. If waxed, peel it. Imported produce is usually highly sprayed, fumigated, and, increasingly, irradiated. They are often used as a substitute for produce that is out of season locally, so buy with caution.

CHAPTER TEN

FOOD PREP 101

If you lead a busy life like I do, you'll want to optimize your time in the kitchen. With a bit of practice, the process of preparing salads, vegetables, and fruits will become quick and easy. Here are some other timesaving tips:

• Cook a healthy "one-pot" meal twice a week.

• Prepare foods in quantity to freeze and eat during the week.

• Purchase fresh, pre-prepped foods.

• Keep a variety of frozen vegetables in the freezer for convenience.

• Use clay pots to prepare dishes in the microwave.

• Use a food processor to chop vegetables.

• Hire a caterer or cook who delivers.

Whatever technique you choose, make sure you eat a variety of raw vegetable salads, cooked vegetables, and fresh and frozen fruits every day. Always have antioxidant-rich foods available to you so they are there when hunger strikes. I always carry a small, insulated bag with an ice pack that is filled with sliced raw vegetables and fruits.

HEALTHY COOKING TECHNIQUES
Steam Sautéing

Steam sautéing is a technique that decreases the loss of antioxidant nutrients. Simply use small amounts of liquid while quickly simmering food over high heat.

Many standard recipes call for sautéing vegetables before making soups and stews. I disagree. My approach is a simple, timesaving one-stage process. In my recipes for soups and stews, I combine the ingredients, add liquid, and simmer until done to my taste.

CLAY POT COOKING

Baking foods in terracotta clay pots is an ancient tradition that dates back to Roman times. Clay pots were soaked in water to create a moist cooking environment for baking in an oven.

I love cooking with clay pots. In fact, I've designated an entire recipe section to this delicious super antioxidant cooking technique. Clay pots are used for a wide variety of dishes, from soups, stews, and vegetable dishes to desserts. They keep food very moist, seal in nutrients, and provide a delightful mix of flavors. They also are perfect for using in the microwave.

Clay pots can be purchased from cookware stores or online. A popular brand is the Romertopf, although there are several excellent brands.

USING A FOOD PROCESSOR

A food processor slashes the time it would otherwise take to chop vegetables by hand. I like to prepare vegetables with different cuts just for variety. You can be creative by experimenting with various techniques and cuts.

NUTTY CREAMED SOUPS

By blending nuts into soups and sauces, you can create dishes that are just as rich and velvety as any cream-based dish. In fact, you might even fool your taste buds with these sinfully delicious but guilt-free recipes.

OTHER TASTY TIPS

You can increase antioxidant power and add taste by:

Topping dishes with foods like:

- chopped nuts, sunflower seeds, lightly toasted ground sesame seeds, and freshly ground flaxseed

- fresh sprouts (especially broccoli sprouts)

- chopped fresh tomatoes, fresh herbs, and/or green onions

- cubed avocado

- Adding finely shredded raw bok choy, Chinese cabbage, romaine lettuce, spinach, kale, grated zucchini, and any other chopped or shredded raw vegetables to your hot soups and stews before serving

- Using fresh vegetable juices in place of water in soups and stews

- Adding raw vegetables, especially leafy greens, when blending hot soups

- Adding raw leafy greens to fruit smoothies

CHAPTER ELEVEN

SUPER ANTIOXIDANT EATING ON THE ROAD

Many people ask me how to stay on the Super Antioxidant Diet while traveling, because most restaurants add loads of fat and sodium to their dishes. Here are some suggestions.

Tasty tips for the road:

- Buy prepackaged fruit and tossed salads to take with you.

- Grab a bag of organic baby spinach. (A bag of spinach, handful of raw nuts or sunflower seeds, and a piece of fruit make a filling meal.)

- Eat a can of beans.

- Eat natural bars that contain only nuts, dates, and fruits. Great picks are LÄRABARs and Cliff Nectar Bars.

- Request a small refrigerator for your hotel room for food storage.

- Take a blender with you (and electric skillet, when possible) for whipping up nutrient-dense dishes in the room.

Wherever you go, search for:

- Stores such as Whole Foods, Wild Oats, or Central Market, where you can buy fresh juices, salads, or prepared meals. Remember to watch the salt and oil!

- Restaurants with salad bars that offer fat-free dressings, balsamic vinegar, lemon juice, or a vinaigrette.

- Juice and smoothie bars.

For restaurant meals:

- Ask for sauces and dressings on the side and use sparingly.

- Ask that your entrée to be prepared without oil or with a reduced amount of oil.

- Order steamed vegetable platters when available.

- Ask for a modified entrée salad.

- For Chinese food, pick steamed mixed vegetables and tofu with sauce on the side.

- In a fast-food restaurant, order green and/or fruit salads.

- If you are not on the Anti-Inflammation Plan, order a baked potato stuffed with fresh salad bar items.

- For breakfast, order oatmeal and fresh fruit, or an egg white and vegetable omelet.

For long trips:

- Order the vegetarian meal on the airplane.

- Prepare or purchase a laminated card of menu preferences (in the appropriate language) to take with you as a reference guide.

After eating the Super Antioxidant Diet for several weeks, you may be tempted to slip back into your old way of eating. Even if you do, don't give up! Just return to healthy eating the next time.

Keeping a weekly diet diary is one way to help you stay your course and know that, occasionally, it's okay to eat whatever you like!

Carry natural whole antioxidant foods with you at all times.

CHAPTER TWELVE

VIBRANT CUISINE MENUS

The Super Antioxidant Diet offers four meal plans. Each plan includes three weeks of daily meal guides and their corresponding recipes. In this book, I have intentionally kept most of my recipes simple and fast, although several gourmet dishes take more time to prepare.

The four Super Antioxidant Diet plans are:

- Meat and Fish Eaters: Limits but allows meat, poultry, fish, and limited dairy products

- Fish Eaters: Includes certain types of fish, but excludes red meat, poultry, or dairy

- The Ultimate Vegan: Includes an abundance of raw vegetables and fruits

- Anti-Inflammation: Limits certain foods

MEAT AND FISH EATERS PLAN

You may include one serving or less of free-range lean meats or wild fish per day on the Meat and Fish Eaters plan. One serving is equal in size to a deck of playing cards. To decrease your risk of certain diseases, consume no more than fourteen ounces[1,2] of lean grass-fed meat, free-range poultry, wild game, or wild fish per week. In this plan, you will be eating an abundance of antioxidant rich vegetables, legumes, fruits, nuts, and seeds for disease protection and health maintenance.

FISH EATERS PLAN

This plan provides you with an abundance of plant foods to give you large amounts of antioxidants for disease protection, as well as several moderate servings of wild fish per week. Keep wild fish consumption to no more than fourteen ounces per week.[3,4]

THE ULTIMATE VEGAN PLAN

Numerous scientific studies show that people who eat a vegan diet (no meat, fish, or dairy) live longer and healthier.[5,6] Our vegan plan will provide the protein, calories, and fat that are required for an average person performing moderate activity. Most important, our plan is packed with antioxidant-rich, whole foods that will provide maximum disease protection and health maintenance. Here are a few important tips to remember:

• Be diligent and careful to follow the recommended guidelines of this plan.

• Take recommended supplements.

• You must take a supplement of vitamin B-12.

• Stay away from the unhealthy natural and organic junk food sold in health food sections. Just because a product says natural, vegan, or organic does not necessarily mean it is healthful. These products are often processed and nutrient deficient.

• Don't overdo nuts, seeds, and dried fruits.

Note: If you wish to follow a raw food diet, be careful. Gradually add raw foods while following the Super Antioxidant Diet's Ultimate Vegan Plan. Once your body has adjusted to this plan, you can probably rather easily transition to a raw food diet.

THE ANTI-INFLAMMATION PLAN

Inflammatory diseases are caused by an overreactive immune system and include arthritis, allergies, asthma, lupus, fibromylalgia, chronic fatigue, gout, atherosclerosis, and diabetes. The major culprit for this overreactive immune system response is the excess production of arachidonic acid, an omega-6 fatty acid. Too much arachidonic acid in the body can cause devastating consequences to the body, which we call inflammation.[7]

Grain-fed animals produce excess amounts of arachidonic acid.[8,9] The acid is found in the fatty tissue of muscle meat, organ meats, and egg yolks. In addition to ingesting the acid in our diets, our bodies produce it when we have high insulin levels.

All of the Super Antioxidant Diet meal plans are designed to combat inflammation, but the Ultimate Vegan Plan and Anti-Inflammation Plan actually work to minimize inflammation. The Bare Minimum Supplements chapter in part 1 discusses a supplement specifically formulated to help combat inflammation.

Arachidonic acid production can be controlled by:

• Eliminating foods that contain large amounts of arachidonic acid such as farm-raised fish, chicken, turkey, and egg yolks. Foods that have very little arachidonic acid are wild fish, free-range chicken, free-range turkey, and wild game. An extra benefit of eating wild salmon is the anti-inflammatory omega-3 fish oil, DHA (docosahexaenoic acid). Organic meats and poultry that are not labeled "free range" or "grass-fed" should be avoided as well.

• Consuming omega-3 and omega-6 in the proper ratio.[10] Research has shown that a ratio of 1:1 of omega-3 and omega-6 is beneficial. Fish oil, flax oil, and borage seed oil are high in omega-3. Lean red meat is high in omega-6 and should be kept to a minimum or avoided alto-

gether.[11] Transformation's Essential Fatty Acids supplement has the proper ratio of 1:1.

• Consuming foods that are low on the glycemic scale. Avoid foods that are processed, contain sugar, or are loaded with trans fats. Processed foods include white flour foods, white rice, and instant oatmeal. Limit sugar-laden foods such as pies, cakes, sweet muffins, candy, and cookies as well as popcorn and crackers. These foods cause an insulin rush and insulin causes the body to produce more arachidonic acid.

• Limiting white potatoes, tomatoes, and eggplant, which are part of the nightshade family. Nightshade vegetables contain a chemical called solanine that can increase inflammation. The Anti-Inflammation Plan contains a limited amount of nightshade vegetables. After reducing or eliminating inflammation, you may add more nightshade vegetables with caution.

CHOOSING MENUS

No matter what plan you choose, consume an *abundance* of whole foods, especially leafy green vegetables. The most antioxidant-rich foods are whole foods in their natural state, but even whole healthy foods, such as raw nuts and seeds, can overload you with fat if eaten in excess. Eating too many dried fruits and dates can also be unhealthy. The only thing you can never eat too much of are *green leafy or colorful vegetables*. I also encourage you to create your own recipes based on the Super Antioxidant Diet guidelines.

TRANSITIONING

If you have trouble adhering to a sudden diet change, you might want to transition to the plan of your choice. During the first week on the diet, try eating the menu of your chosen plan *for only one day*. During the second week, abide by your plan for two days, and so on. By the seventh week, you will have completely transitioned to the Super Antioxidant Diet.

If you find that you don't have time to follow the menus, just remember to eat:

1. Two or more cups of a variety of fresh or frozen cooked vegetables (include 1 cup or more cruciferous vegetables)

2. Three to five different fresh or frozen fruits (including blueberries)

3. Half a cup to one-and-a-half cups cooked legumes (dried cooked beans)

4. Three cups or more tossed salad with leafy greens and raw vegetables

5. One ounce raw nuts and/or seeds

6. Half a cup to one cup whole grains

7. Optional: Two to four ounces lean grass-fed meat, free-range poultry, free-range egg whites, wild game, or wild-caught fish (four times per week or fewer)

MENU COMPARISONS

Following are sample menus for three of the four diets. I've excluded the Anti-Inflammation Plan because its foods are similar to the Fish Eaters Plan. Recipes for these plans are included in the recipe section.

MENU COMPARISON ONE

Meat and Fish Eaters Sample Menu	Fish Eaters Sample Menu	Ultimate Vegan Sample Menu
BREAKFAST Fruity Oatmeal • Orange Juice	BREAKFAST Fruit and Berry Smoothie	BREAKFAST Low-Glycemic Smoothie
LUNCH Navy Bean Salad Niçoise • Curried Tomato Bisque • Seeded Flat Bread Crackers	LUNCH Tuscan Vegetable Lentil Soup • Pineapple and Blueberry Compote	LUNCH Middle-Eastern Salad Platter • ¼ cup Hummus Dip • Handful of Nuts • Fresh Fruit of Choice
DINNER Baked Blueberry-Garlic Chicken • Roasted Vegetables • Tossed Green Salad • Fruit and Berry Compote	DINNER Wild Flounder Florentine • Brown Rice • Tossed Salad w/ Chopped Veggies and Tahini Dressing • Pomegranate Poached Pear w/ Berry-Berry Sauce	DINNER Antioxidant Thai Vegetable Curry • Steamed Brown Rice • Tropical Fruit Plate (Mango, Papaya, Kiwi)
Total Calories: 1,782 Total Fat: 38 grams Calories from Fat: 22% Protein: 64 grams	Total Calories: 1,757 Total Fat: 41 grams Calories from Fat: 20% Protein: 66 grams	Total Calories: 1,700 Total Fat: 41 grams Calories from Fat: 22.2% Protein: 58 grams

Now let's compare the preceding Super Antioxidant Diets with sample menus of three typical American diets (see chart on next page). Anything look familiar?

MENU COMPARISON TWO

Fast-Food Suicide Sample Menu	Gourmet Suicide Sample Menu	Faux Healthy Sample Menu
BREAKFAST	BREAKFAST	BREAKFAST
Blueberry Muffin	Eggs Benedict • Mixed Fruit • Cappuccino	Low-Fat Yogurt w/ Fruit • Blueberry Muffin • Orange Juice
LUNCH	LUNCH	LUNCH
Fast-Food Big Bacon Classic Hamburger • Super-sized French Fries • Diet Cola • Brownie	Bouillabaise (French Fish Stew) • French Baguette w/ Butter	Caesar Salad with 3 oz Grilled Chicken • Apple • 2 oz String Cheese
DINNER	DINNER	DINNER
Chicken Pasta Alfredo w/ Broccoli • Salad w/ Ranch Dressing • French Bread w/ Olive Oil • Ice Cream	Roast Duckling • Turnip Puree • Green Beans w/ Browned Butter • Romaine Salad w/ Vinaigrette • French Baguette w/ Butter • Brie Cheese and Fruit	Grilled Farm-Raised Salmon • Small Baked Potato • 1 tsp Butter • 2 oz Light Sour Cream • ½ cup Steamed Broccoli • ½ cup Granola • 4 oz Frozen Yogurt
Total Calories: 3,382 Total Fat: 206 grams Calories from Fat: 54% Protein: 109 grams	Total Calories: 4,980 Total Fat: 368 grams Calories from Fat: 67% Protein: 180 grams	Total Calories: 2,381 Total Fat: 115 grams Calories from Fat: 43% Protein: 130 grams

NUTRITIONAL VALUE COMPARISON
OF SAMPLE MENUS

	FAST-FOOD SUICIDE	GOURMET SUICIDE	FAUX HEALTHY	MEAT AND FISH EATERS	FISH EATERS	ULTIMATE VEGAN
Calories	3,382	4,980	2,381	1,703	1,757	1,708
Total Fat (g)	206	368	115	39	41	42
Saturated Fat	67	133	30	6	6	6
Monosaturated Fat (g)	59	169	20	21	16	13
Polyunsaturated Fat (g)	19	42	17	10	13	7
Cholesterol (mg)	396	1,295	290	77	54	0
Carbohydrate (g)	283	225	212	277	311	300
Dietary Fiber (g)	17	22	20	58	45	57
Protein (g)	109	180	130	81	66	61
Sodium (mg)	4,502	6,336	3,043	1,320	560	610
Potassium (mg)	995	4,915	3,880	5,885	6,096	5,437
Calcium (mg)	7	889	1,408	881	753	1,002
Iron (mg)	4	34	11	30	23	32
Zinc (mg)	4	18	9	10	10	10
Vitamin C (mg)	46	211	151	524	361	593
Vitamin A (IU)	2,676	13,576	4,335	57,154	56,673	74,535
Vitamin B-6 (mg)	9	2.9	3.4	3.3	3.4	2.6
Vitamin B-12 (mcg)	1.4	11.9	9.8	.4	1.8	0
Thiamin B-1 (mg)	1.0	3.7	1.5	1.9	2.1	1.8
Riboflavin B-2 (mg	.9	3.8	1.9	1.3	1.7	1.5
Folacin (mcg)	117	448	372	1,072	780	882
Niacin	22	50	32	29	20	16

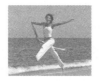

CHAPTER THIRTEEN

VIBRANT CUISINE MEAL GUIDES

Recipes for the dishes in italics can be found in chapter 14.

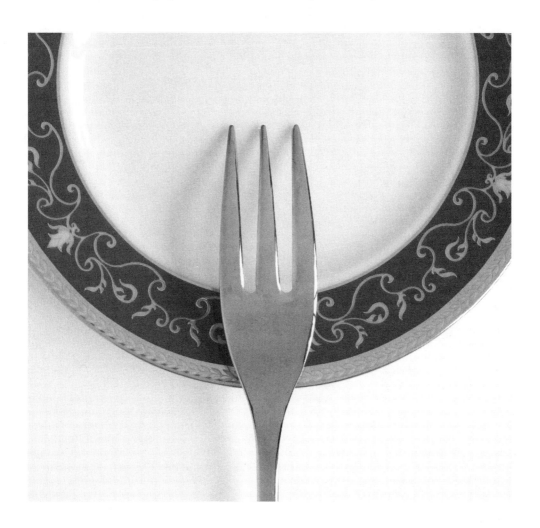

MEAT AND FISH EATER'S PLAN: WEEK ONE

DAY	Breakfast	Lunch	Dinner
1	Bowl of fresh fruit • 1 slice preservative-free whole-grain toast with 1 tbsp casher butter and fruit juice-sweetened fruit spread	Tuscan Chopped Salad • Fresh fruit	Tomato-Topped Wild Salmon on Asparagus and Spinach • Green salad with fruit
2	Low-Glycemic Green Fruit Smoothie	Leftover Salmon Veggie Wrap • Split Pea, Leek, and Kale Soup • Fresh fruit	Rotisserie Chicken Salad • Ginger Squash Soup
3	Perfect Porridge	Fast Italian Tomato-Bean Soup • Robin's Favorite Chopped Salad • Fresh fruit	Carrot-Chicken Stir-Fry • Brown Rice • Chocolate Divine Mousse Ice Cream
4	Fresh fruit sprinkled with unsweetened granola and a dollop of fat-free plain yogurt (add 2 tsp dehydrated date sugar to sweeten)	Petra Chopped Salad • Fresh fruit	African Ground-Nut Chicken-Okra Stew • Pear Walnut Salad with Pomegranate Vinaigrette
5	Rise-and-Shine Juice • 1 slice whole-grain preservative-free toast with goat or sheep cheese and sliced tomato	Quick Garlic-Broccoli Bean Soup • Green salad with dressing of your choice • Fresh fruit	Baked Wild Snapper Florentine with Artichokes and Tomatoes • Garlic Lemon Spinach • Tropical Fruit Compote
6	Cherry-Banana Romaine Smoothie	Leftover Quick Garlic Broccoli Bean Soup • Classic Middle Eastern Hummus Dip with raw vegetables	Sweet Potato–Vegetable Pie • Pinky Chopped Salad • Robin's Very Berry Creamy Ice Cream
7	Swiss Muesli	Essene Chopped Salad • Fresh fruit	Citrus Wild Salmon with Garlic Greens • Tracy's Cashew-Peanut Stew

MEAT AND FISH EATER'S PLAN: WEEK TWO

DAY	Breakfast	Lunch	Dinner
1	Perfect Porridge	Rotisserie Chicken-Apple Salad • Summer Fresh Gazpacho • Fresh fruit	Quick Vegetable-Bean Chili • Confetti Salad • Fresh berries
2	Fresh fruit sprinkled with unsweetened granola and a dollop of fat-free plain yogurt (add 2 tsp dehydrated date sugar to sweeten	Green salad • Leftover Vegetable-Bean Chili • Fresh fruit	Grilled or Sauteed Chicken Breast with Portobello Mushroom Stew and Broccoli in Orange Sauce • Simple Chocolate-Nut Dip with fresh strawberries and fruit
3	Hot Cinnamon-Fruit Oatmeal	Tuscan Chopped Salad	Asisan-Mexican Fusion Stir-Fry • Brown rice • Green salad • Fresh fruit
4	Peachy-Green Smoothie	Split Pea, Leek, and Kale Soup • Cilantro Hummus Dip with raw vegetables	Indian Vegetable Chicken Curry • Brown rice • Vibrant Asparagus, Bean, and Mushroom Salad
5	Rise-and-Shine Juice • 1 slice whole-grain preservative-free toast with goat or sheep cheese and sliced tomato	Leftover Split Pea, Leek and Kale Soup • Chopped salad of your choice • Fresh or frozen berries	Baked Blueberry-Garlic Chicken Breast • Baked Aromatic Spice and Butternut Squash • Green Salad
6	Blueberry-Orange Smoothie	Veggie Wrap • Refreshing Watermelon Gazpacho	Large green salad with dressing of your choice • Tuscan-Baked Squash with Tomato-Vegetable-Bean Sauce • Fresh fruit
7	Breakfast Burrito	Vibrant Fruit Salad with Cherry-Berry Dressing	Wild Salmon Chowder Confetti Salad • 6 preservative-free whole-grain crackers • Fresh fruit

MEAT AND FISH EATER'S PLAN: WEEK THREE

DAY	Breakfast	Lunch	Dinner
1	Tropical Smoothie	Southwestern Corn-Asparagus Soup • 6 preservative-free whole-grain crackers • Cilantro Hummus Dip with raw vegetables	Basic Grilled Salmon • Roasted Vegetables • Tuscan Kale–Mushroom Sauté • Fresh fruit
2	Swiss Muesli	Rotisserie Chicken Salad • Cup of leftover Southwestern Corn-Asparagus Soup	Easy Stuffed Eggplant or Cabbage Rolls • Vegetable Mashed Sweet Potatoes • Vibrant Asparagus, Bean, and Mushroom Salad • Creamy Fruit Compote
3	Smoothie of your choice	Southwestern Avocado-Bean Wrap	Wild Salmon Salad Niçoise • Pomegranate-Poached Pears with Cherry-Berry Sauce
4	Rise-and-Shine Juice • 1 slice whole-grain preserverative-free toast with 1 tbsp cashew butter and fruit juice-sweetened fruit spread	Savory Vegetable Bean Soup • Green salad with your choice of dressing • Fresh fruit	Bison Fillets with Mushroom-Pepper Wine Sauce • Cashew Mashed Cauliflower with Leeks and Mushrooms • Confetti Salad
5	Perfect Porridge	Ginger Squash Soup • Pear-Walnut Salad with Pomegranate Vinaigrette	Carrot-Citrus Chicken • Vegetable Mashed Sweet Potatoes • Green salad with fruit
6	Breakfast Salad	Pronto Black Bean Vegetable Soup • Petra Chopped Salad	Vegetable Pizza • Leftover soup • Fresh fruit
7	Creamy Carob-Banana Smoothie	Vegetable Rotini Soup • 6 preservative-free whole-grain crackers	Garlic Chicken and Collards Stir-Fry • Chopped salad of your choice • Baked Fruit Delight

FISH EATER'S PLAN: WEEK ONE

DAY	Breakfast	Lunch	Dinner
1	Green Gulp Smoothie	Pronto Black Bean Vegetable Soup • Salad • Fresh fruit	Antioxidant Lasagna • Large green and raw vegetable salad • Fresh fruit
2	Low-Glycemic Green Fruit Smoothie	Large chopped salad of your choice • Fresh fruit	Stovetop Ratatouille • Autumn Harvest Stuffed Winter Squash • Confetti Salad • Chocolate Divine Mousse Ice Cream
3	Hot Cinnamon-Fruit Oatmeal	Vibrant Fruit Salad with Cherry-Berry Dressing • Cancer-Defense Juice	Easy Stuffed Eggplant • Creamy Kale with Mushrooms and Onions • Tossed mixed salad with your choice of dressing • Fresh fruit
4	Cherry-Berry Muesli	Petra Chopped Salad • Fresh fruit	Pecan-Encrusted Salmon • Roasted Vegetables • Salad of your choice • Fresh fruit
5	Low-Glycemic Green Fruit Smoothie	Fast Italian Tomato-Bean Soup • Curried Hummus Dip with raw vegetables • Fresh fruit	Basic Grilled Salmon with Mango Pineapple Salsa • Cashew Mashed Cauliflower with Leeks and Mushrooms • Green salad • Pomegranate Poached Pears with Cherry-Berry Sauce
6	Green Gulp Smoothie	Leftover Fast Italian Tomato-Bean Soup • Salad of your choice	Large green salad • Anti-oxidant Juice • Chipotle Hummus Dip with raw vegetables • Fresh fruit
7	Perfect Porridge • Cancer-Defense Juice	Eclectic Chopped Salad with Citrus-Cashew Dressing	Sake Steamed Wild Salmon w/ Ginger Sauce • Baked sweet potato • Fresh fruit

FISH EATER'S PLAN: WEEK TWO

DAY	Breakfast	Lunch	Dinner
1	Fresh fruit • Whole-grain toast with 1 tbsp raw nut butter	Spinach Pea Soup • Eagle-Eye Salad	Vegetable Strata with Tomato Salsa • Green salad • Tropical Fruit Parfaits
2	Smoothie of your choice	Athenian Chopped Salad • Cancer-Defense Juice	African Ground-Nut Vegetable Stew • Confetti Salad • Fresh or frozen cherries
3	Swiss Muesli Cereal	Leftover African Ground-Nut Vegetable Stew • Roasted Portobello Salad • Cancer-Defense Juice	Antioxidant Lasagna • Mixed greens and raw vegetable salad • Fresh or frozen berries
4	Perfect Porridge	Ginger Squash Soup • Your choice of green salad • Fresh fruit	Wild Salmon and Asparagus Green Curry • Steamed brown rice • Fresh fruit
5	Fresh fruit with fat-free plain yogurt and raw nuts	Tofu-Vegetable Chili • Green salad • Fresh fruit	Stuffed Bell Peppers • Cashew Mashed Cauliflower with Leeks and Mushrooms • Baked Fruit Delight
6	Green Gulp Smoothie	Leftover Tofu-Vegetable Chili • Salad • Antioxidant Juice	Large green salad with dressing of your choice • Tuscan-Baked Squash with Tomato-Vegetable-Bean Sauce • Fresh fruit
7	Big-C Smoothie	Leftovers • Fresh fruit	Curried Lentil Soup • Tossed green salad with fruit

FISH EATER'S PLAN: WEEK THREE

DAY	Breakfast	Lunch	Dinner
1	Green Gulp Smoothie	White Gazpacho • Essene Chopped Salad	Tuscan-Baked Squash with Tomato-Vegetable-Bean Sauce • Broccoli with Currants and Pine Nuts • Chocolate Dip with fresh fruit and berries
2	Swiss Muesli	Fast Italian Tomato-Bean Soup • Eclectic Chopped Salad with Citrus-Cashew Dressing	Grilled Rainbow Trout with Roasted Vegetables • Large tossed green salad with your choice of dressing • Fresh fruit
3	Smoothie of your choice	Vibrant Fruit Salad with Cherry-Berry Dressing	Asian-Mexican Fusion Stir-Fry • Brown rice • Fresh fruit
4	Perfect Porridge	Leftover Fast Italian Tomato-Bean Soup • Chopped salad of your choice	Gazpacho of your choice • Antioxidant Juice • Baked Fruit Delight
5	Swiss Muesli	Ginger Squash Soup • Pear-Walnut Salad with Pomegranate Vinaigrette	Pecan-Encrusted Salmon • Vegetable Mashed Sweet Potatoes • Green salad
6	Whole-grain toast with almond butter and banana	Pronto Black Bean Vegetable Soup • Robin's Favorite Chopped Salad	Vegetable Pizza • Leftover soup of your choice • Fresh fruit
7	Low-Glycemic Green Fruit Smoothie	Leftover Pronto Black Bean Vegetable Soup • Cottage Tofu Lettuce Wraps • Granny Smith apple	Vibrant Asparagus, Bean, and Mushroom Salad • Chocolate Jubilee Pudding Cake

THE ULTIMATE VEGAN PLAN: WEEK ONE

DAY	Breakfast	Lunch	Dinner
1	Low-Glycemic Green Fruit Smoothie	Tuscan Chopped Salad—large serving	Antioxidant Lasagna • Large salad • Fresh fruit
2	Fresh fruit and nuts	Green Gazpacho • Creamy Fruit Compote	Pinky Chopped Salad • Steamed Broccoli-Garlic-Red Bell Pepper Medley
3	Hot Cinnamon-Fruit Oatmeal	Vibrant Fruit Salad with Cherry-Berry Dressing • Cancer-Defense Juice	Creamy Kale with Mushrooms and Onions • Robin's Favorite Chopped Salad • Chocolate Divine Mousse Ice Cream
4	Citrus-Goji Smoothie	Power-Boost Gazpacho • Cancer-Defense Juice	Fast Italian Tomato-Bean Soup • Mixed green salad with fruit and choice of dressing
5	Swiss-Miss Green Smoothie	Leftover Fast Italian Tomato-Bean Soup • Antioxidant Juice	Cottage Tofu Lettuce Wraps • White Gazpacho
6	Breakfast Burrito	Special Chili Beans • Green salad with chopped vegetables	Vibrant Asparagus, Bean, and Mushroom Salad • Fresh fruit
7	Perfect Porridge • Cancer-Defense Juice	Eclectic Chopped Salad with Citrus-Cashew Dressing • Fresh fruit	Antioxidant Thai Vegetable Curry • Brown rice • Chopped mixed salad • Fresh fruit

THE ULTIMATE VEGAN PLAN: WEEK TWO

DAY	Breakfast	Lunch	Dinner
1	Low-Glycemic Green Fruit Smoothie	Curried Hummus Dip with raw vegetables • Create your own vegetable juice	Tuscan-Baked Squash with Tomato-Vegetable-Bean Sauce • Green salad with fruit and your choice of dressing
2	Perfect Porridge	Hearty Gazpacho • Whole-grain bread with raw nut butter	Curried Lentil Soup • Petra Chopped Salad • Fresh fruit
3	Swiss Muesli	High-Octane Smoothie	Tracey's Cashew-Peanut Stew • Cashew Mashed Cauliflower with Leeks and Mushrooms • Essene Chopped Salad
4	Peachy-Green Smoothie	Pronto Black Bean • Vegetable Soup • Cancer-Defense Juice	Asian-Mexican Fusion Stir-Fry • Large baby greens salad with choice of dressing
5	Big-C Smoothie	Romaine Banana-Strawberry-Cashew Wrap • Green Gazpacho	Athenian Chopped Salad • Fresh fruit
6	Green Gulp Smoothie	Leftover Pronto Black Bean Vegetable Soup • Pear-Walnut Salad with Pomegranate Vinaigrette	Ginger Squash Soup • Chocolate Divine Mousse Ice Cream
7	Citrus-Goji Smoothie	Cottage Tofu Lettuce Wraps • Summer Fresh Gazpacho	Curried Lentil Soup • Fresh fruit

THE ULTIMATE VEGAN PLAN: WEEK THREE

DAY	Breakfast	Lunch	Dinner
1	Low-Glycemic Green Fruit Smoothie	Petra Chopped Salad— large serving	Antioxidant Lasagna • Large salad • Fresh fruit
2	Cherry-Berry Muesli	Green Gazpacho • Creamy Fruit Compote	Tuscan Chopped Salad • Steamed Broccoli-Garlic-Red Bell Pepper Medley
3	Bowl of fresh fruit • 1 slice preservative-free whole-grain toast or ½ slice bagel with cashew butter and 100% Fruit Spread	Vibrant Fruit Salad with Cherry-Berry Dressing • Cancer-Defense Juice	Creamy Kale with Mushrooms and Onions • Robin's Favorite Chopped Salad • Fresh fruit
4	Citrus-Goji Smoothie	Power-Boost Gazpacho • Cancer-Defense Juice	Fast Italian Tomato-Bean Soup • Mixed green salad with fruit and choice of dressing
5	Breakfast Burrito	Leftover Fast Italian Tomato-Bean Soup • Antioxidant Juice	Cottage Tofu Lettuce Wraps • White Gazpacho
6	Green Gulp Smoothie	Special Chili Beans • Green salad with chopped vegetables	Pinky Chopped Salad • Fresh fruit
7	Perfect Porridge • Cancer-Defense Juice	Eclectic Chopped Salad with Citrus-Cashew Dressing	Antioxidant Thai Vegetable Curry • Brown rice • Chopped mixed salad • Chocolate Divine Mousse Ice Cream

ANTI-INFLAMATION PLAN: WEEK ONE

DAY	Breakfast	Lunch	Dinner
1	Bowl of fresh fruit • 1 slice preservative-free whole-grain toast with cashew butter and 100% Fruit Spread	Tuscan Chopped Salad • Fresh fruit	Tomato-Topped Wild Salmon on Asparagus and Spinach • Tossed green salad with fresh berries
2	Low-Glycemic Green Fruit Smoothie	Savory Salmon Veggie Wrap • Vegetable-Bean Soup • Fresh fruit	Vegetable Chicken Soup with Basil-Garlic Pistou • Green salad with raw veggies and broccoli sprouts
3	Perfect Porridge	Fast Italian Tomato-Bean Soup • Robin's Favorite Chopped Salad	Broiled Orange Wild Salmon • Red Cabbage–Apple Slaw with Cider Yogurt Dressing • Fresh fruit
4	Fresh fruit sprinkled with unsweetened granola and a dollop of fat-free plain yogurt (add 2 tsp dehydrated date sugar to sweeten)	Petra Chopped Salad • Fresh fruit	African Ground-Nut Chicken-Okra Stew • Pear-Walnut Salad with Pomegranate Vinaigrette
5	Rise-and-Shine Juice • 1 slice whole-grain preservative-free toast with goat or sheep cheese and sliced tomato	Quick Garlic-Broccoli Bean Soup • Green salad with choice of dressing • Fresh fruit	Pecan-Encrusted Baked Salmon • Belgian Endive–Fennel Salad with Orange Vinaigrette • Tropical Fruit Compote
6	Low-Glycemic Green Fruit Smoothie	Leftover soup • Classic Curried Hummus Dip with raw vegetables	Sweet Potato–Vegetable Pie • Your choice of chopped veggie salad
7	Swiss Muesli	Chopped veggie salad of your choice—large serving	Citrus Wild Salmon with Garlic Greens • Asian Mixed Vegetables

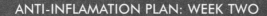

ANTI-INFLAMATION PLAN: WEEK TWO

DAY	Breakfast	Lunch	Dinner
1	Perfect Porridge • Fresh or frozen berries	Very Wild Salmon Salad • Fresh fruit	Tuscan-Baked Squash with Tomato-Vegetable-Bean Sauce • Green salad with fruit and your choice of dressing
2	Whole-grain toast with 1 tbsp almond butter • Fresh fruit	Quick Veggie Citrus Chopped Salad—large serving	Chicken Breasts with Leek-and-Mushroom Stuffing • Roasted Fennel • Tossed green salad • Fresh fruit
3	Swiss Muesli	High-Octane Smoothie	Fast Italian Tomato-Bean Soup • Mixed green salad with fruit and choice of dressing
4	Low-Glycemic Green Fruit Smoothie	Pronto Black Bean Vegetable Soup • Cancer-Defense Juice	Pecan-Encrusted Salmon • Large baby greens salad with broccoli sprouts and choice of dressing
5	Hot Cinnamon-Fruit Oatmeal	Romaine Banana-Strawberry-Cashew Wrap • Green Gazpacho	Wild Salmon with Sesame-Orange-Ginger Relish over Braised Bok Choy • Baked sweet potato
6	Breakfast Burrito • Fresh berries	Leftover Pronto Black Bean Vegetable Soup • Pear-Walnut Salad with Pomegranate Vinaigrette	Ginger Squash Soup • Fresh fruit
7	Perfect Porridge	Cottage Tofu Lettuce Wraps • Summer Fresh Gazpacho	Wild Salmon Patties with Fresh Tomato Salsa • Lemony Green Beans and Pine Nuts • Fresh fruit

ANTI-INFLAMATION PLAN: WEEK THREE

DAY	Breakfast	Lunch	Dinner
1	Smoothie of your choice	Gazpacho of your choice • Whole-grain bread with 1 tbsp nut butter • Fresh fruit	Grilled Salmon and Bean Salad • Fresh fruit
2	Swiss Muesli	Split-Pea, Leek, and Kale Soup • Eclectic Chopped Salad with Citrus-Cashew Dressing	Smokey Venison Vegetable Goulash • Belgian Endive–Fennel Salad
3	Hot Cinnamon-Fruit Oatmeal • Cancer-Defense Juice	Vibrant Fruit Salad with Cherry-Berry Dressing	Steamed Broccoli-Garlic-Red Bell Pepper Medley • Tuscan-Baked Squash with Tomato-Vegetable-Bean Sauce • Simple Chocolate-Nut Dip with fresh fruit and berries
4	Low-Glycemic Green Fruit Smoothie	Leftover Smokey Venison Vegetable Goulash • Chopped salad of your choice	Gazpacho of choice • Antioxidant Juice • Pomegranate-Poached Pears with Cherry-Berry Sauce
5	Perfect Porridge	Ginger Squash Soup • Pear-Walnut Salad with Pomegranate Vinaigrette	Wild Salmon Packages with Fennel, Sweet Potatoes, Leeks, and Olives • Fresh fruit
6	Smoothie of your choice	Pronto Black Bean Vegetable Soup • Athenian Chopped Salad	Red Cabbage–Blueberry-Apple Slaw with Cider-Yogurt Dressing • Leftover Pronto Black Bean Vegetable Soup • Fresh fruit
7	Breakfast Salad	Southwestern Corn-Asparagus Soup • Granny Smith apple	Basic Grilled Salmon Broccoli with Currants and Pine Nuts • Chocolate Jubilee Pudding Cake

CHAPTER FOURTEEN

ROBIN'S VIBRANT CUISINE RECIPES

BREAKFASTS
Smoothies

When we chew our food, only a small percentage of nutrients in the food is released into the bloodstream. By blending fruits and vegetables, we dramatically increase our nutrient absorption. Smoothies are very beneficial for the elderly and people who have trouble absorbing nutrients.

Blueberries are included in several smoothie recipes because of their high antioxidant content. I also recommend adding pomegranate juice and Acai berry juice because they are very high in antioxidants.

To make your smoothies more antioxidant rich, use one or two leaves of raw kale, bok choy, or leafy lettuce (not iceberg) in addition to spinach or romaine. The fiber in raw kale is difficult for some people to digest; try a small amount to see how it works for you. If you have no problem with it, gradually increase the amount you use. Since leafy greens are loaded with antioxidants, the more you add to your smoothie the quicker you will improve your health! As you become accustomed to more greens, add broccoli and other cruciferous vegetables for an antioxidant boost.

A good way to get your daily omega-3 is to add flaxseeds to your breakfast smoothie. Simply grind flaxseeds in a coffee grinder or in the bottom of a dry blender. Grind enough for the week and store it in the freezer for easy use.

Use the Vibrant Cuisine smoothie while learning how to create your nutrient-loaded drinks. You can omit soy milk, and use almond milk, juice, or water instead, and any fruit and leafy green combination you desire. Using frozen fruit makes a smoothie-freeze.

Because nutrients like natural fruit sugar are extremely absorbable, it is recommended you limit smoothies to three or four times a week. Diabetics, after getting approval from their doctors to adopt the Super Antioxidant Diet, should avoid the smoothies until their blood sugar drops to normal levels without medication. To reduce glycemic levels, reduce fruit while adding more greens. Liquefying leafy greens makes it easier and more practical for you to consume the amount you need for adequate nutrition.

Unlike all other diet programs, the key to the Super Antioxidant Diet is to consume enough of the right foods. You can drink some of your smoothies and refrigerate the rest to drink throughout the day. Be sure to blend your smoothie on high for one to two minutes until it is very smooth.

LOW-GLYCEMIC GREEN FRUIT SMOOTHIE
Servings: 1–2

¼ cup pomegranate juice or Acai juice (Acai juice is lower in natural sugars than pomegranate juice. Both items can be found in health food stores and some supermarkets.)

½ to 1 cup water or unsweetened soy milk

6 romaine lettuce leaves or 2 to 3 ounces organic spinach

2 kale leaves, de-stemmed

1 orange, peeled, seeded, and separated in half

2 cups frozen blueberries

2 tablespoons freshly ground flaxseed

1 teaspoon cinnamon—optional (helps to lower blood sugar)

Blend liquid, lettuce or spinach, and kale until smooth (about 1 minute). Add remaining ingredients and blend until smooth and creamy. If you suffer from arthritis add one teaspoon ground turmeric.

CHERRY-BERRY SMOOTHIE
Servings: 2

3 handfuls fresh baby spinach, washed

½ cup soy milk

½ cup pomegranate juice (or another unsweetened fruit juice)

½ cup water

1 medium banana

1 cup frozen blueberries

1 cup frozen cherries

1 orange, peeled and seeded, leaving some of the white

1 kiwi, peeled

4 tablespoons freshly ground
   flaxseed

Blend spinach, soy milk, pomegranate juice, and water first to liquefy the spinach, then add other ingredients and blend until smooth and creamy.

CHERRY-BANANA-
ROMAINE SMOOTHIE
Servings: 2

½ cup pomegranate or Acai juice
½ cup water or soy milk
5 to 6 large romaine leaves
1 cup frozen cherries
1 cup blueberries
1 banana
4 tablespoons freshly ground
   flaxseed

Blend liquid and romaine first. Add remaining ingredients and blend until smooth. Add water if necessary.

PEACHY-GREEN SMOOTHIE
Servings: 2

½ cup pomegranate juice
1 cup water
1 to 2 handfuls of spinach leaves
1 cup ice
3 ripe peaches

1 banana
4 tablespoons freshly ground
   flaxseed

Blend liquid and spinach first. Add remaining ingredients and blend until smooth.

BLUEBERRY-ORANGE SMOOTHIE
Servings: 2

½ cup water
3 dates
1 banana
2 whole oranges, peeled and seeded
1 cup frozen blueberries
2 tablespoon freshly ground
   flaxseed

Blend until smooth.

TROPICAL SMOOTHIE
Servings: 2

1 cup papaya, cubed
½ cup pineapple chunks (fresh or
   frozen)
1 kiwi, peeled and cubed
¼ cup coconut milk
½ cup mango, cubed
1 cup ice
½ cup pineapple juice
4 tablespoons freshly ground
   flaxseed

Blend all ingredients until smooth. This smoothie is even better when you use frozen fruit. Just omit the ice and add water or more juice if needed.

CREAMY CAROB-BANANA SMOOTHIE
Servings: 2

1 cup frozen strawberries or
   blueberries
1 banana
2 tablespoons carob powder
½ cup pomegranate juice
½ cup unsweetened soy milk
4 tablespoons freshly ground
   flaxseed

Blend until smooth.

CHOCOLATE DREAM SMOOTHIE
Servings: 2

3 ounces fresh spinach
½ cup soy, rice, or almond milk
½ cup pomegranate juice
½ cup water
1 medium banana
1–3 tablespoons cocoa powder
1 cup frozen mixed fruit
1 cup frozen blueberries

2 tablespoons freshly ground
   flaxseed

Blend spinach and liquids first. Add remaining ingredients and blend until smooth. If too thick, add more water as necessary.

Note: Cocoa powder is derived from beans that contain large quantities of natural antioxidants. There have been numerous scientific studies that show the benefits of consuming the antioxidants contained in cocoa. Only use natural cocoa powder, not Dutch processed. Most supermarkets carry natural cocoa powder in their baking section.

GREEN GULP SMOOTHIE
Servings: 2

1 whole orange, peeled and seeded
3 to 4 handfuls baby spinach
3 leaves kale
½ cup orange or pineapple juice
½ cup water
1 kiwi, peeled
1 cup honeydew melon, cubed
1 cup frozen pineapple chunks
1 banana
4 tablespoons freshly ground
   flaxseed

Blend orange, spinach, kale, juice, and water until liquefied. Add remaining ingredients, blending until smooth and creamy. Add more water or juice if needed.

MEGA-C SMOOTHIE
(High in vitamin C)
Servings: 2

½ cup water
½ cup orange juice
½ cup pomegranate juice
1 handful baby spinach leaves
3 to 4 large chard leaves
1 cup frozen strawberries
2 oranges, peeled and seeded,
    leaving white
2 ripe kiwis, peeled
1 ripe banana
3 pitted dates
½ cup raw broccoli florets
4 tablespoons freshly ground
    flaxseed

Blend liquid, spinach, and chard until liquefied. Add remaining ingredients and blend until smooth. Add more liquid if necessary.

GINGER-MINT FLIP SMOOTHIE
Servings: 2

½ cup water
½ cup carrot juice

½ cup pomegranate juice
2 cups baby spinach leaves
2 kale leaves
10 mint leaves
1 cup frozen pineapple chunks
1 banana
1 thin slice fresh ginger
2 tablespoons freshly ground
    flaxseed

Blend liquid, spinach, kale, and mint until liquefied. Add remaining ingredients and blend until smooth.

CITRUS-GOJI SMOOTHIE
Servings: 2

½ cup pomegranate juice
½ cup orange juice
½ cup water
5 ounces (1 bag) organic baby
    spinach
½ cup frozen blueberries
1 medium orange, peeled and
    seeded, leaving the white
1 kiwi, peeled
¼ cup goji berries (can be
    purchased in some health
    food stores or online)
1 whole banana (optional)
2 tablespoons freshly ground
    flaxseed

Blend liquids and spinach until liquefied. Add remaining ingredients

and blend until smooth and
creamy.

SWISS-MISS GREEN SMOOTHIE
Servings: 2

½ cup water
½ cup pomegranate juice
½ cup unsweetened soy milk
  (optional)
4 large Swiss chard leaves
1 large mango
1 cup mixed frozen fruit
1 banana
2 tablespoons freshly ground
  flaxseed

Blend liquid and chard first.
Add remaining ingredients and
blend until smooth.

HIGH-OCTANE SMOOTHIE
(For athletes or those
wanting to gain weight)
Servings: 1

½ cup pomegranate juice
½ cup soy, almond, or rice milk
4 handfuls baby spinach
2 leaves of kale, stems removed
1 cup frozen blueberries
3 tablespoons goji berries
½ avocado
24 raw cashews
1 banana

2 tablespoons freshly ground
  flaxseed

Blend liquid with spinach and
kale until liquefied. Add remaining
ingredients and blend until smooth.
Add more juice as necessary.

Cereals

SWISS MUESLI CEREAL
Servings: 2

½ cup pomegranate juice
½ cup water
½ cup steel cut or rolled oats (not
  quick-cooking oats)
2 tablespoons currants
1 whole Granny Smith apple,
  grated
1 banana, sliced
1 cup of halved grapes
½ cup cubed cantaloupe
½ cup sliced strawberries
1 cup blueberries
4 tablespoons freshly ground
  flaxseed
3 tablespoons chopped raw nuts
3 tablespoons nonfat plain yogurt
  or soy yogurt (optional)

Soak oats in pomegranate juice
and water overnight in refrigerator.

Oats will absorb all liquid. Combine all ingredients and mix.

You may add any fruits. The original Swiss Muesli served at Dr. Bircher's famous Swiss health clinic mixed in plain yogurt. If you choose, add nonfat plain yogurt or soy yogurt.

CHERRY-BERRY MUESLI
Servings: 2

½ cup oats
½ cup pomegranate juice
1 banana, sliced
1 cup blueberries (fresh or frozen and thawed)
1 cup pitted cherries (fresh or frozen and thawed)
1 Granny Smith apple, chopped
4 tablespoons freshly ground flaxseed
¼ cup soy, rice, or almond milk
3 tablespoons nonfat plain or soy yogurt (optional)
2 tablespoons chopped raw nuts

Soak oats overnight in pomegranate juice. Add other ingredients, mix, and serve.

HOT CINNAMON-FRUIT OATMEAL
Servings: 2

½ cup old-fashioned rolled oats
2 cups water
¼ teaspoon cinnamon
1 cup frozen blueberries
½ cup frozen mixed fruit
1 whole Granny Smith apple, grated
¼ cup currants or raisins
2 tablespoons chopped walnuts
4 tablespoons freshly ground flaxseed

In a saucepan, combine water, oats, and cinnamon and bring to a boil over high heat. Reduce the heat and simmer until oats are cooked. Add blueberries and fruit and simmer until berries are heated through. Remove from heat. Mix in apples, currants or raisins, nuts, and flaxseed. Add more cinnamon if you like. Stir and serve.

PERFECT PORRIDGE
Servings: 6

½ cup chopped fresh or frozen broccoli
½ cup chopped zucchini
1 cup chopped bok choy or cabbage
2 cups water or broth

1 cup old-fashioned rolled oats

6 tablespoons freshly ground
flaxseed

2 tablespoons nutritional yeast

6 tablespoons sunflower seeds

3 teaspoons Bragg Liquid Amino
Acids (or to taste)

Simmer vegetables in water or
broth until almost tender. Add oatmeal and simmer to desired consistency and vegetables are tender.
Remove from heat. Add flaxseed
and yeast. Serve sprinkled with
sunflower seeds and Bragg to taste.

BREAKFAST SALAD
Servings: 4

2 cups romaine lettuce and/or
spinach, shredded and coarsely
chopped

1 orange, peeled, seeded, and
segmented

2/3 cup papaya, cubed

1 cup grape halves

1 cup fresh or frozen blueberries

1/2 cup halved strawberries

1 apple, grated

1 kiwi, cubed

1/2 cup raw oatmeal

2/3 cups pomegranate juice

6 tablespoons freshly ground
flaxseed

1/4 cup goji berries or currants

Assorted mixed raw nuts

Toss all ingredients and serve
topped with raw nuts.

Note: You can make this with
any assortment of fruits.

BREAKFAST BURRITO
Servings: 6

1/2 cup red bell pepper, seeded and
finely chopped

3 green onions, diced

2 cloves garlic, minced or pressed

1/3 cup water

2 cups red or black beans

1 1/2 teaspoons Bragg Liquid Amino
Acids

1 medium tomato, chopped

Any salt-free herb seasoning, to
taste

3 tablespoons nutritional yeast (or
to taste)

5 ounces (1 bag) organic baby
spinach, coarsely chopped
(optional)

6 tablespoons freshly ground
flaxseed

1/4 cup grated soy cheese

Ezekiel Sprouted Grain Tortillas

In a large skillet, sauté bell pepper, onion, and garlic in 1/3 cup
water for 5 minutes. Add the beans

and Bragg, cooking for another 5 minutes. Remove from heat and mix in tomatoes, seasoning, yeast, spinach (if using), flaxseed, and soy cheese. Lightly toast the tortillas and stuff with bean filling.

Note: This also makes a great hot or cold sandwich filling for wraps or stuffed in a whole-wheat pita.

KAREN'S RAINBOW OMELET
Servings: 2

½ ounce porcini dried mushrooms
½ medium red onion, diced
½ red bell pepper, seeded and diced
½ yellow bell pepper, seeded and diced
½ medium zucchini, diced
2 teaspoons Bragg Amino Acids
1 tablespoon balsamic vinegar (to taste)
olive oil spray
½ cup Egg Beaters or egg whites, halved
2 tablespoons shredded soy cheese

Place porcini mushrooms in a small glass bowl and cover with water. Microwave for 1 minute and set aside until ready to use (can also heat on stove until tender).

Place onions, red bell pepper, yellow bell pepper, zucchini, mushrooms, Bragg, and balsamic vinegar in a wok and steam-sauté for about 5 minutes on medium heat.

Scoop all ingredients from wok, leaving the liquid. Reduce liquid until thickened and sauce-like. After liquid is reduced, set aside in a bowl and use as sauce for vegetables on omelet.

In omelet skillet, spray small amount of olive oil and prepare omelet using ¼ cup Egg Beaters or egg whites per omelet. After turning omelet, put 1 tablespoon of shredded soy cheese in middle of omelet with ¼ of sautéed vegetables. Fold omelet and put on plate, and top with ¼ more vegetables. Drizzle sauce over omelet and serve.

Juices and Drinks

Be creative and come up with your own juice blends.

ARISE-AND-SHINE
JUICE (Blender)
Servings: 2

1 cup mini carrots
2 cups fresh pineapple, or 20-ounce

can unsweetened pineapple, with juice
⅛ organic lemon with rind
1 teaspoon grated fresh ginger (optional)
1 tablespoon goji berries (optional)

Combine all ingredients in a blender and blend until smooth. To make this more like a juice, add 2 cups of ice before blending. This is a refreshing and vibrant drink.

WATERMELON SLUSH (Blender)
Servings: 2

4 to 6 cups cubed watermelon
1 teaspoon raspberry vinegar

In blender, liquefy until smooth. You can add some ice if you like.

BOMBAY CANTALOUPE LASSI (Blender)
Servings: 4

4 cups cubed cantaloupe
1 cup nonfat kefir or nonfat yogurt
mint for garnish (optional)

Place cantaloupe and yogurt in a blender and blend until smooth. Garnish with mint.

CANCER-DEFENSE JUICE (Juicer)
Servings: 2

6 cauliflower florets
½ head broccoli with stems
2 cups watercress
8 kale leaves
6 medium carrots
2 whole apples

Juice all ingredients in a juicer and drink.

ANTIOXIDANT JUICE (Juicer)
Servings: 1–2

8 carrots
2 beets
3 kale leaves
2 bok choy leaves
½ head cauliflower
½-inch slice of fresh ginger

Juice all ingredients and drink.

UNEXPECTED DELIGHT JUICE (Blender)
Servings: 2

1 cup unsweetened pineapple juice
1 cup water
1 cup frozen pineapple chunks
1 cup cubed cantaloupe
1 raw carrot

4 kale leaves, stripped from stems
1 kiwi, peeled and sliced
1 tablespoon freshly ground
   flaxseed

Combine in a blender and blend until smooth.

STEAMED TEA DRINK
Servings: 1

$2/3$ cup water
$1/3$ cup soy milk
1 green, rooibos, or other herbal
   tea bag
½ teaspoon honey

Heat water and soy milk. Pour into a mug. Steep tea bag in the hot liquid for 3 minutes and add honey. Delicious!

Note: This is my favorite drink. I make it with Tazo Calm tea as a winding-down drink. You can request this from any café that serves steamed soy milk. Just tell them how it is prepared. Rooibos chai tea is delicious prepared this way. Remember to keep your honey consumption under 1 teaspoon per day.

REFRESHING ANTIOXIDANT TEA PUNCH WITH FRUIT
Servings: 8 (12 ounces each)

1 quart water
6 Tazo Passion tea bags
6 rooibos tea bags
1 quart pomegranate cherry juice
1 nectarine, peeled (if not organic)
   and quartered
1 organic orange cut into quarter-
   inch rounds
1 cup blueberries
8 sprigs of fresh mint, crushed

Bring water to a boil, remove from heat, add tea bags, and let steep for 10 minutes. Remove tea bags and add pomegranate cherry juice, fruit, and mint. Serve in glass pitcher with ice.

SALADS

TOSSED GREEN SALAD WITH SEEDS AND FRUIT
Servings: 4

2 cups baby salad mix
2 cups romaine torn or cut into
   bite-sized pieces
2 cups watercress
1 cup broccoli sprouts
2 tablespoons sunflower seeds

...pples, chopped
...liced strawberries
...espoons currants
...blespoon rice vinegar
2 ...ablespoons orange juice
2 teaspoons cold-pressed olive oil
2 teaspoons Bragg Liquid Amino
Acids
¼ cup raw sunflower seeds
¼ cup raw pumpkin seeds
2 tablespoons unhulled sesame
seeds

Toss all ingredients together
except for sesame seeds. Top with
sprinkled seeds and serve.

Note: You can lightly toast
seeds in a dry skillet until they just
begin to turn light brown.

ROTISSERIE CHICKEN SALAD
Servings: 4

2 cooked chicken breasts (store-
bought free-range rotisserie
chicken), shredded
1 head of romaine lettuce, shredded
2 tomatoes, chopped
1 avocado, cubed
10 black olives
1 sweet onion, thinly sliced
1 raw carrot, shredded
1 cucumber, cubed
3 tablespoons water
3 tablespoons tahini

1 tablespoon cider vinegar
3 teaspoons Bragg Liquid Amino
Acids
1 small garlic clove, pressed
½ teaspoon ground cumin

Toss all ingredients and serve.

VIBRANT ASPARAGUS, BEAN, AND MUSHROOM SALAD
Servings: 6

2 bunches fresh asparagus
1 red bell pepper, seeded and sliced
in thin strips
½ pound shiitake mushrooms,
stems removed and sliced (¼-
inch thickness)
½ pound white mushrooms, sliced
6 cloves garlic, pressed
¼ cube Rapunzel Salt-Free
Bouillon (optional)
2 cups cooked beans (cannellini,
pinto, black, or red)
½ cup chopped parsley
2 teaspoons cold-pressed olive oil
2 teaspoons Bragg Liquid Amino
Acids
¼ cup pine nuts

To remove woody ends from
asparagus, take hold of an asparagus spear at both ends, and bend
the spear until it breaks. The place
it breaks is where the "woodiness"

begins. Take the one broken asparagus, line it up next to the bunch, and cut the whole bunch at the same place. Cut the asparagus on the diagonal in 1½ inch pieces. Blanch asparagus for 2 to 3 minutes in boiling water. In colander, rinse with cold water.

Steam-sauté the pepper, mushrooms, garlic, and bouillon for 5 to 8 minutes until peppers are soft. Gently toss together asparagus, mushroom mix, beans, half the chopped parsley, olive oil, and Bragg. Serve sprinkled with remaining parsley and pine nuts.

CONFETTI SALAD
Servings: 4

2 cups romaine lettuce, shredded
2 cups mache (a cruciferous leafy green, available at many large supermarkets)
2 cups baby salad mix
2 cups baby arugula
1 cup watercress sprigs
½ cup fresh blackberries
½ cup fresh raspberries
½ cup fresh blueberries
½ cup fresh strawberries
½ cup sweet onion—thinly sliced
½ cup edible marigold flower petals (found in the fresh herb section of some stores)

Dressing

2 teaspoons Bragg Liquid Amino Acids
2 tablespoons balsamic vinegar
2 teaspoons honey
1 small garlic clove, pressed
2 teaspoons cold-pressed olive oil

In large salad bowl, toss salad greens with dressing. Sprinkle with berries, onion, and flower petals.

Note: You can use any green salad mix.

PEAR-WALNUT SALAD WITH POMEGRANATE VINAIGRETTE
Servings: 4

1 cup pomegranate juice
1 shallot, sliced
2 tablespoons cold-pressed olive oil
2 tablespoons red wine vinegar
1 small clove garlic, pressed
12 cups mixed baby greens
½ cup raw walnut halves
3 ripe pears cut into ½-inch slices (you can use apples)

For dressing, bring pomegranate juice and shallot to boil in saucepan. Reduce heat to medium-low, and simmer until reduced to about ½ cup. Remove from heat. Whisk in oil, vinegar, and garlic.

Toss greens, walnuts, and pears in dressing, and serve.

CRISP GREEN SALAD
Servings: 4

10 cups mixed baby greens of your
  choice
2 cups arugula
1 cup broccoli sprouts
1 carrot, grated
½ sweet onion, thinly sliced

Toss in dressing of your choice.

ROASTED PORTOBELLO SALAD
Servings: 4

4 large portobello mushrooms,
  stems removed
Olive oil spray
1 teaspoon Bragg Liquid Amino
  Acids
6 cloves garlic, minced (or 2
  teaspoons powdered garlic)
5 handfuls baby mixed greens
5 handfuls baby spinach
2 cups watercress sprigs
2 cups chopped tomatoes
1 cup sliced cucumber
1 red bell pepper, seeded and
  chopped
2 (15-ounce) cans garbanzo beans,
  drained

½ cup chopped green onions
1 zucchini, grated
1 carrot, grated

Dressing

3 tablespoons tahini
2 teaspoons Bragg Liquid Amino
  Acids
1 tablespoon lemon juice
1 clove garlic, minced
¼ cup water
½ teaspoon cumin

Preheat oven to 350 degrees. Lightly oil two baking sheets. Place portobello caps on baking sheet. Mix garlic and Bragg. Spray caps with olive oil and spread with garlic and Bragg mixture. Bake 10 minutes until tender and slightly browned.

Whisk dressing. If too thick, add more water. Assemble all salad ingredients and toss with dressing. Top with warm roasted mushrooms.

VIBRANT FRUIT SALAD WITH CHERRY-BERRY DRESSING
This is a full meal! Be creative and use any combination of fruits.
Servings: 8

8 cups shredded romaine lettuce
½ cup chopped celery

2 kiwis, peeled, quartered, and
  sliced
1 pint fresh strawberries, quartered
1 apple cut into 1-inch cubes
1 banana, sliced
½ cup currants or goji berries
2 oranges, peeled, sliced, and
  seeded
2 ounces chopped pecans

Dressing

1 cup frozen mixed blueberries and
  strawberries, thawed
1 cup frozen pitted cherries,
  thawed
½ cup raw cashews
2 tablespoons rice vinegar
2 teaspoons organic orange zest
  (made before peeling the orange,
  or you can peel one strip from
  the orange and toss it in the
  blender to make zest)
1 medium organic orange, peeled
  and seeded, leaving white part
½ cup orange juice
½ cup pomegranate juice

Puree all dressing ingredients in
blender until smooth. Taste and
correct seasoning if necessary. It
should be tart and sweet. Toss
ingredients except for orange slices
and pecans in dressing. Place
orange slices on salad and sprinkle
with chopped pecans.

EAGLE-EYE SALAD
Servings: 4

5 whole carrots, shredded
1 cup halved grapes
2 kiwis, peeled and sliced
4 cups shredded romaine
½ sweet onion, coarsely chopped
½ cup sliced strawberries
½ cup orange juice
½ cup carrot juice
2 tablespoons cashew butter
1 tablespoon minced fresh dill or 1
  teaspoon dried
1 tablespoon raspberry vinegar
½ teaspoon Bragg Liquid Amino Acids
Any salt-free herb seasoning, to taste
¼ cup coarsely chopped raw
  cashews

In large mixing bowl, combine
carrots, grapes, kiwis, and romaine.
In blender, blend onion, strawberries, juices, cashew butter, dill, vinegar, Bragg, and seasoning and blend
until smooth. Pour dressing over
carrots, fruit, and romaine mixture
and toss. Sprinkle with cashews.

ROMAINE-FRUIT-CASHEW WRAP
Servings: 1

1 to 2 tablespoons cashew butter
8 or more large romaine leaves,
  washed and dried

1 banana, sliced
1 apple, sliced
6 strawberries, halved

Spread cashew butter on romaine leaf. Place banana slices, apple slices, and strawberry halves on cashew butter and roll leaf.
Note: You can use any fruit.

BELGIUM ENDIVE–FENNEL SALAD WITH ORANGE VINAIGRETTE
Servings: 4

2 organic navel oranges
1½ tablespoons wine vinegar
1 teaspoon Bragg Liquid Amino Acids
3 teaspoons cold-pressed olive oil
2 medium fennel bulbs (sometimes called anise, 2 pounds total), stalks discarded
2 whole Belgian endives, trimmed
½ cup coarsely chopped walnuts

Finely grate enough zest from orange to measure 2 teaspoons, and then squeeze 1 tablespoon orange juice into a large bowl. Whisk in zest, vinegar, Bragg, and oil until combined well. Cut fennel bulbs lengthwise into very thin slices. Halve endives lengthwise, then halve crosswise, and cut lengthwise into ¼-inch-wide strips. Add

endive and fennel to vinaigrette and toss to combine. Chill covered for 15 minutes to allow flavors to develop. Serve topped with walnuts.

COTTAGE-TOFU LETTUCE WRAPS
Servings: 4

1 pound firm or extra-firm tofu, drained and mashed
3 tablespoons raw tahini
2 tablespoons lemon juice
1 clove garlic, minced
2 teaspoons miso
1 tablespoon chopped fresh tarragon
¼ cup chopped green onions
½ cup grated carrots
½ cup cubed tomatoes
1 cup chopped broccoli
1 cup broccoli sprouts
16 leaf lettuce or raw collard green leaves, washed and dried

Mix all ingredients, except leaves, to make filling. Fill lettuce leaves with all ingredients, roll, and wrap.

RED CABBAGE–APPLE SLAW WITH CIDER-YOGURT DRESSING
Servings: 3

½ medium head red cabbage (about 1 pound)

1 large fennel bulb (sometimes
   called anise, about 1 pound)
½ sweet onion, sliced very thinly
½ English cucumber, ¼-inch dice
2 Granny Smith apples
1 cup fresh blueberries
3 tablespoons slivered almonds,
   lightly toasted

Dressing

¾ cup clear apple cider or apple juice
¾ cup plain nonfat yogurt
2 tablespoons chopped fresh parsley
2 tablespoons finely chopped fresh dill
1 teaspoon Bragg Liquid Amino
   Acids

Halve cabbage lengthwise, and with a sharp knife cut crosswise into very thin shreds. Trim fennel stalks flush with bulb, discarding stalks, cut fennel, and dice to ¼-inch pieces.

For dressing, boil cider or juice in a small saucepan until reduced to about 3 tablespoons, about 15 minutes. Cool cider or juice slightly and in a bowl whisk together with yogurt, parsley, dill, and Bragg.

Just before serving, coarsely chop apples and add with blueberries to other salad ingredients. Toss with dressing and serve topped with almonds.

CHOPPED SALADS

Chopped salads contain everything you need for a complete meal. They are a delicious way to prepare an assortment of raw live vegetables so that each mouthful is saturated with a flavorful nutritious dressing. Mound dressed salad on dinner plates and top with sprouts and seeds or nuts for an impressive presentation. With each bite, your taste buds delight and your body rejoices!

Take any combination of chopped or grated non-starchy vegetables and combine them with thinly shredded romaine lettuce and cabbage. Try the following recipes. Create your own using any of the dressing recipes or your own concoctions. I recommend that when you make a dressing, make plenty to have on hand in the refrigerator. You can also stretch a homemade dressing by adding some natural commercial dressing (check the label for unhealthy ingredients).

ROBIN'S FAVORITE CHOPPED SALAD
Servings: 3

1 medium romaine lettuce, washed, dried, and shredded

1 whole red bell pepper, seeded and chopped

1½ cups cooked or canned red kidney beans

3 stalks celery, chopped

¼ whole sweet onion, thinly sliced

1 medium cucumber, cubed

2 cups cherry or grape tomato halves

1 broccoli stalk with crown, chopped

1 carrot, grated

1 small zucchini, grated

1 medium avocado, cubed

2 tablespoons hemp seeds (purchased in health food store or some supermarkets—optional)

¼ cup raw sunflower seeds

1 cup broccoli sprouts

Spicy Tahini Dressing

1 clove garlic, peeled and chopped

½ teaspoon cumin

¼ teaspoon chili powder

4 tablespoons tahini (pureed sesame seeds)

2 teaspoons Bragg Liquid Amino Acids

½ cup water

¼ cup cider vinegar

Place dressing ingredients in blender or bowl. Blend or whisk until smooth. Sauce should be the consistency of heavy cream. If too thick, add more water and lemon juice. In large bowl, toss all salad ingredients with dressing except sunflower seeds and sprouts. Mound on dinner plates, sprinkle with sunflower seeds, top with sprouts, and serve.

QUICK VEGGIE CITRUS CHOPPED SALAD
Servings: 4

1 cup shredded romaine lettuce

2 cups halved cherry tomatoes

3 cups cooked lentils or 2 (15-ounce) cans, drained

2 whole avocados, cubed

4 medium carrots, grated

½ cup raw sunflower seeds

½ cup chopped green onions

2 whole red bell peppers, seeded and thinly sliced

4 oranges, peeled, sliced, and seeded, or tangerine segments

½ cup fat-free raspberry dressing (store-bought)

1 teaspoon Bragg Liquid Amino Acids

12 ounces mixed baby greens

3 tablespoons chopped walnuts

Toss all ingredients with dressing except for baby greens and walnuts. Make a bed of baby greens on dinner plates. Pile tossed mixture on top of greens and sprinkle with walnuts.

ATHENIAN CHOPPED SALAD
Servings: 3

1 medium romaine lettuce, washed, dried, and shredded
1 whole red bell pepper, seeded and chopped
2 cups cooked or canned garbanzo beans
12 kalamata olives, rinsed
3 stalks celery, chopped
¼ whole sweet onion, thinly sliced
1 medium zucchini, grated
½ medium cucumber, cubed
1 medium tomato, cubed, or ½ cup halved grape or cherry tomatoes
1 medium avocado, cubed

Combine all salad ingredients, and toss thoroughly with Middle Eastern Tahini Dressing (recipe in Dressings, Sauces, and Dips section) and serve.

ESSENE CHOPPED SALAD
Servings: 4

5 ounces baby organic spinach
3 cups shredded romaine lettuce
4 mushrooms, thinly sliced
1 small sweet onion, thinly sliced
2 medium tomatoes, chopped
1 medium cucumber, chopped

1 medium red bell pepper, seeded and chopped
4 tablespoons sesame seeds

Eggplant Hummus Dressing

1 eggplant
1 cup cooked or canned garbanzo beans
3 tablespoons tahini
3 tablespoons lemon juice
5 cloves garlic, chopped fine
⅓ cup bean liquid (from the can of garbanzo beans) or water
1 teaspoon Bragg Liquid Amino Acids

Prick eggplant and bake on baking sheet at 350 degrees for 45 minutes. Scoop out eggplant meat. In a blender or food processor combine eggplant, garbanzo beans, tahini, lemon juice, garlic, bean liquid, and Bragg. Blend until smooth. Using half of the eggplant hummus, toss with salad ingredients, and sprinkle with sesame seeds. Save remaining eggplant hummus for a raw vegetable dip.

TUSCAN CHOPPED SALAD
Servings: 4

2 (15-ounce) cans navy beans, unsalted, drained

1 cup chopped celery, medium fine
½ cup chopped red bell pepper,
  medium fine and seeds removed
½ cup shredded carrots
¼ cup chopped walnuts
1 cup chopped plum tomato
¼ cup chopped scallion
½ cup fresh parsley
3 cups shredded romaine lettuce

Quick Piquant Dressing

3 tablespoons raw cashew or
  almond butter
1 cup tomato pasta sauce (lowest in
  sodium you can find)
3 tablespoons balsamic vinegar
1 teaspoon garlic powder
1 tablespoon Spike Salt-Free
  Seasoning
3 teaspoons Bragg Liquid Amino
  Acids

Whisk dressing together until
smooth. Thoroughly toss all ingredients and serve mounded on a dinner plate.

PETRA CHOPPED SALAD
Servings: 4

1 large head romaine lettuce,
  chopped
1 medium cucumber, cubed
½ sweet onion, thinly sliced
2 cups frozen peas, thawed

1 medium tomato, diced
1 red bell pepper, seeded and
  chopped
2 tablespoons currants
¼ cup slivered almonds, lightly
  toasted if you like
¼ cup raw sunflower seeds
2 cups (salt-free) garbanzo beans

Dressing

2 tablespoons cold-pressed olive oil
2 tablespoons balsamic vinegar
½ teaspoon Bragg Liquid Amino
  Acids
2 teaspoons garlic powder

Place all salad ingredients in large
salad bowl. Whip dressing together,
toss with salad, and serve. Add more
balsamic vinegar if you like.

PINKY CHOPPED SALAD
Servings: 4

4 handfuls salad greens—combination of mache, baby greens, baby
  spinach, curly endive, watercress
1 cup thinly shredded red cabbage
3 cups shredded romaine lettuce
1 cup grated carrots
½ cup grated raw beets
1 avocado, cubed
10 cherry or grape tomatoes, halved
½ cup broccoli sprouts
½ cup raw unsalted pistachio nuts

Light Dressing

2 teaspoons Bragg Liquid Amino
  Acids
2 teaspoons cold-pressed olive oil
1 tablespoon rice vinegar
¼ teaspoon garlic powder
1 teaspoon Dijon mustard
½ cup sesame seeds

Lightly toast a cup of sesame seeds (preferably with hulls) in dry skillet until they begin to brown and pop. Quickly remove from the stove and grind in dry blender or coffee grinder. Store in freezer to use as a calcium-rich, tasty topping for soups, salads, main dishes, and more.

In large mixing bowl, place all salad ingredients except for sprouts and nuts. Whisk together all dressing ingredients except sesame seeds. Toss salad with light dressing and top with sprouts, ground seeds, and nuts.

ECLECTIC CHOPPED SALAD WITH CITRUS-CASHEW DRESSING
Servings: 4

4 cups shredded romaine lettuce
1 cup watercress
¼ cup dried unsweetened cherries
2 kiwis, sliced

½ cup coarsely chopped walnuts
1 cup orange sections, seeded
1 cup sliced strawberries
½ cup sesame seeds, lightly toasted

Dressing

1 medium orange, peeled and
  seeded
1 small key lime or ½ regular lime,
  peeled and seeded
1 tablespoon raspberry vinegar
¼ cup orange juice
½ teaspoon orange zest (from
  organic orange)
¼ cup raw cashews and blanched
  almonds

Assemble salad ingredients, except sesame seeds. Blend all dressing ingredients until smooth and creamy. Add more orange juice to thin if needed. Toss all ingredients and sprinkle with sesame seeds.

DRESSINGS, SAUCES, AND DIPS

Many of the sauces are nut and seed based. As well as being rich and delicious, they are loaded with nutrients. You may substitute any raw nut butter of your choice. These creamy dressings are delicious as dips for raw vegetables.

SPICY CHIPOTLE-MAPLE VINAIGRETTE
Yield: 1¾ cups

1½ cups orange juice
2 teaspoons maple syrup
1 tablespoon cold-pressed virgin olive oil
1 tablespoon finely chopped red onion
1 teaspoon fresh lime juice
1 teaspoon chopped canned chipotle chili in adobo sauce, plus 1 teaspoon of the sauce
2 teaspoons Bragg Liquid Amino Acids

Whisk together all ingredients until well combined. Toss with salad.

SESAME CARROT DRESSING
Yield: 6

1 tablespoon raw cashew butter
⅔ cup plus 2 tablespoons sesame seeds, lightly toasted
½ clove garlic
7 pitted dates, or to taste
1 cup carrot juice
2 tablespoons seasoned rice vinegar
1 teaspoon toasted sesame oil
soy milk, for thinning

Place all ingredients except for 2 tablespoons sesame seeds in a blender and blend until smooth and creamy. Stir in remaining sesame seeds. Add soy milk to thin if needed.

CITRUS GINGER DRESSING
Yield: ¾ cup

½ cup fresh orange juice
2 tablespoons balsamic vinegar
2 tablespoons natural peanut butter
1 teaspoon toasted sesame oil
2 teaspoons Bragg Liquid Amino Acids
½ garlic clove, minced or pressed
1 chunk fresh ginger (approximately the size of ½ a thumb), peeled

Place all ingredients in blender and blend until smooth and creamy.

GREEN SUPREME DRESSING
Yield: 3 cups

2 cloves garlic, peeled and chopped
1 cup navy beans
8 ounces silken tofu
4 teaspoons Bragg Liquid Amino Acids
1 cup water
½ cup fresh lemon juice
¼ cup chopped parsley
2 cups fresh spinach

Combine all ingredients in blender and blend until smooth. Sauce should be the consistency of heavy cream. If too thick, add more water or lemon juice.

This makes a great dip.

EASY TOMATO-NUT DRESSING
Yield: 1¼ cups

1 cup tomato pasta sauce
½ cup raw almonds
1 tablespoon balsamic vinegar
1 clove garlic, cut in half
3 teaspoons Bragg Liquid Amino Acids
2 teaspoons Spike Salt-Free Seasoning

Combine all ingredients in blender and blend until smooth and creamy. Add additional seasonings if you like.

CITRUS-CASHEW DRESSING
Yield: 2 cups

1 organic orange, peeled and seeded
1 small key lime or ½ regular lime, peeled and seeded
1½ by 1-inch strip of organic orange peel
½ cup fresh or frozen pineapple chunks

2 tablespoons rice vinegar
½ cup orange juice
¼ cup raw cashews

Combine all ingredients in a blender and blend until smooth and creamy. Add more orange juice to thin if necessary. Add additional vinegar to suit your taste.

SUNNY MUSTARD DRESSING
Yield: 1½ cups

½ cup lightly toasted sunflower seeds
3 tablespoons lemon juice
¼ teaspoon garlic powder
1 teaspoon Dijon mustard
1 tablespoon freshly ground flaxseed
1 teaspoon Bragg Liquid Amino Acids
¾ cup water

Place all ingredients in blender and blend until smooth and creamy.

MIDDLE EASTERN TAHINI DRESSING OR SAUCE
Yield: 2 cups

2 cloves garlic, chopped
½ cup tahini
2 teaspoons balsamic vinegar

4 teaspoons Bragg Liquid Amino
  Acids
1 pinch crushed red pepper
juice of 1 lemon
½ teaspoon paprika
¼ cup lightly packed fresh parsley
½ cup cold water

Place all ingredients in blender
and blend until smooth and creamy.

THAI-STYLE PEANUT SAUCE
Yield: ⅔ cup

2 whole oranges, peeled and seeded
3 tablespoons seasoned rice vinegar
1 tablespoon unsalted peanut
  butter
1 tablespoon raw cashew butter
1 clove garlic, minced
1 teaspoon grated ginger root
1 tablespoon chopped fresh basil
¼ cup cilantro
2 whole dates
¼ teaspoon red pepper flakes
1 teaspoon Bragg Liquid Amino
  Acids
orange juice (optional)

In a blender or food processor,
combine the ingredients and blend
until smooth. Adjust the seasonings and serve. If you prefer a thin-
ner dressing, add orange juice until
dressing reaches desired consistency.

HEARTY MIXED MUSHROOM SAUCE
Yield: approximately 4 cups

1 large onion, chopped
1 red bell pepper, seeded and thinly
  sliced
2 teaspoons chopped fresh rosemary
2 teaspoons Bragg Liquid Amino
  Acids
2 pinches of red pepper flakes
1 pound large white mushrooms,
  thickly sliced
½ pound shiitake mushrooms,
  sliced
¼ cup dried porcini mushrooms,
  rehydrated (optional)
2 garlic cloves, minced
3 tablespoons tomato paste
1¼ cups mushroom stock or water
¼ cup white wine
2 teaspoons Worcestershire sauce
1 teaspoon balsamic vinegar
2 tablespoons chopped fresh parsley
  or tarragon

Steam-sauté the onion, bell pepper, and rosemary, stirring occasionally until tender, about 8
minutes. Add Bragg and red pepper
flakes. Add the mushrooms and
sauté until tender and juicy, about 5
minutes. Add the garlic, tomato paste,
stock, wine, Worcestershire, and
vinegar. Simmer gently, uncovered,

for 12 to 15 minutes. Remove from heat. Add the parsley.

CLASSIC MIDDLE EASTERN HUMMUS DIP
Yield: 2½ cups

2 cups cooked or canned garbanzo
  beans, drained
3 to 4 cloves garlic
¼ cup fresh lemon juice
¼ cup water
¼ cup raw tahini
½ teaspoon ground cumin
pinch cayenne pepper
pinch of sea salt to taste

In food processor, place the garbanzo beans, garlic, lemon juice, and water. Pulse a few times. Then scrape down the sides of the bowl and continue processing until pureed. If very thick, add a little water to thin. Add the tahini, cumin, cayenne, and salt and pulse until well combined. Serve with raw vegetables.

CHIPOTLE HUMMUS DIP
Yield: 2½ cups

3 to 4 cloves garlic
2 cups cooked or canned garbanzo
  beans, drained
¼ cup cider vinegar
¼ cup water
¼ cup raw almond butter
1 minced chipotle plus 1 tablespoon sauce (from a can of
  chipotle chilies in adobo sauce)
½ teaspoon chili powder
pinch of sea salt to taste
½ cup chopped roasted red peppers
  (you can use jar variety)

In food processor, combine the garlic, garbanzo beans, vinegar, and water, and pulse a few times. Scrape down the sides of the bowl and continue processing until pureed. If very thick, add a little water to thin. Add almond butter, chipotle, adobo sauce, chili powder, and salt and pulse until well combined. Stir in roasted red peppers. Serve with raw vegetables.

CURRIED HUMMUS DIP
Yield: 2½ cups

2 cups cooked or canned garbanzo
  beans, drained
3 to 4 cloves garlic, minced
¼ cup lemon juice
¼ cup water
¼ cup raw cashew butter
2 tablespoons curry powder
½ cup currants
pinch of sea salt to taste

In food processor, combine garlic, garbanzo beans, lemon juice, and water, and pulse a few times. Add cashew butter and curry powder, and pulse until well combined. Scrape down the sides of the bowl and continue processing until pureed. If very thick, add a little water to thin. Fold in currants and season with a little salt. Serve with raw vegetables.

CILANTRO HUMMUS DIP
Yield: 2½ cups

2 cups cooked or canned garbanzo
   beans, drained
3 to 4 cloves garlic, minced
¼ cup rice vinegar
¼ cup water
⅛ cup unsalted peanut butter
⅛ cup raw almond butter
½ cup lightly packed chopped fresh
   cilantro leaves
1 teaspoon toasted sesame oil
2 teaspoons Bragg Liquid Amino
   Acids

In food processor, add the garlic, garbanzo beans, rice vinegar, and water, and pulse a few times. Scrape down the sides of the bowl and continue processing until pureed. If very thick, add a little

water to thin. Add peanut butter, almond butter, cilantro, sesame oil, and Bragg and then pulse until well combined. Serve with raw vegetables.

MANGO-PINEAPPLE SALSA
Yield: 3 cups

1 cup, peeled, pitted, and chopped
1 cup chopped pineapple
1 cup chopped red bell pepper,
   seeds removed
⅔ cup chopped green onions
¼ cup chopped fresh cilantro
2 tablespoons fresh lime juice

Mix all ingredients in small bowl.
Note: This can be made 6 hours ahead. Cover and chill.

FRESH TOMATO SALSA
Yield: 2 cups

2 whole tomatoes, coarsely
   chopped
1 onion, chopped
1 clove garlic
½ jalapeño chili pepper, seeded and
   minced
3 tablespoons chopped cilantro
3 tablespoons fresh lime juice
1 teaspoon Bragg Liquid Amino
   Acids

In a mixing bowl, combine all ingredients. Serve or refrigerate in a tightly covered container for up to 3 days.

PINEAPPLE-PEACH SALSA WITH FRESH MINT
(for Grilled Salmon)
Yield: 2½ cups

1 cup fresh pineapple, cut into ½-inch pieces
1 cup fresh peach, cut into ½-inch pieces
1 sweet onion, coarsely chopped
1 clove garlic, pressed
juice of 1 lime
½ cup coarsely chopped fresh mint

Gently toss ingredients and serve with salmon.

SOUPS

BASIC COOKED BEANS
Servings: 6

1 pound (2 cups) uncooked beans, your choice
6 cups water, for soaking
6 cups water, for cooking
1 large onion, cut in quarters
8 cloves garlic, peeled and sliced
Salt-free seasonings, your choice
(for red beans, black, or pinto, I like chili powder and cumin)
1 or 2 sheets dried sea vegetable (kombu, hiziki, wakame, or dulse—optional)

Soak beans in 6 cups water for 8 hours or overnight. Rinse and drain beans. Place beans, onion, garlic, seasonings, and sea vegetable (if used) in a large pot and cover with 6 cups fresh water, or to about one inch above the beans. Cover and gently simmer until tender when taste-tasted, 1½ to 2 hours. Add hot water as needed to keep beans just covered with liquid.

Keep in the refrigerator to accompany vegetables, add to salads, soups, and vegetable dishes, or eat as is. Eating beans accompanied by raw vegetables or salads can decrease gas. Beans can be frozen for later use.

Note: After soaking beans, if you find you do not have time to cook them, simply rinse, drain, and freeze until ready to use.

BASIC LENTILS
Servings: 6

2 cups lentils (green, red, or French)
5 cups water

1 onion, cut in quarters
10 cloves garlic, peeled and sliced

Lentils do not have to be soaked. Rinse and drain lentils. Place lentils, onion, and garlic in a large pot with 5 cups water, or to about one inch above the lentils. Cover and gently simmer until tender when taste-tasted, 30 to 45 minutes. Red lentils take about 30 minutes.

Keep in the refrigerator to accompany vegetables, add to salads, soups, and vegetable dishes, or eat as is. They can be frozen for later use.

GINGER SQUASH SOUP
Servings: 8

3 cups cubed butternut squash or 1 can pumpkin puree
1 cup sliced carrots
1 cup thinly sliced onion
1 clove garlic
3 tablespoons chopped ginger
4 cups water
3 teaspoons Bragg Liquid Amino Acids
¼ cube Rapunzel Salt-Free Bouillon (sold in health food stores)
½ teaspoon organic orange zest
⅔ cup raw cashews

4 oranges, peeled and seeded
1 cup soy or almond milk
10 ounces fresh baby spinach
1 teaspoon snipped fresh parsley

In covered saucepan, heat the first 8 ingredients to boiling. Reduce heat; simmer, covered, 30 minutes or until squash is tender. Puree the mixture. You will have to do it in batches. In the final batch, add zest, cashews, oranges, and almond or soy milk and blend until smooth. Return the whole pureed mixture to pot and stir well. Heat pureed mixture. Add spinach and stir until just wilted, then serve, garnished with parsley.

FAST ITALIAN TOMATO-BEAN SOUP
Servings: 10

4 cups prepared natural or organic tomato soup (found in health food stores)
4 cups frozen spinach
4 cups frozen chopped broccoli
1 cup fresh or frozen chopped onions
2 cups frozen peas
1 can (15 ounces) diced tomatoes (lowest sodium)

1 or 2 sheets dried sea vegetable
(kombu, hiziki, wakame, or
dulse—optional)
3 cups carrot juice
2 teaspoons garlic powder
2 teaspoons dried Italian herbs
4 cans (15 ounces each) salt-free
red beans
4 tablespoons pine nuts or walnuts

In a large pot, combine all
ingredients except beans and nuts
and simmer for 40 minutes. Add
beans and simmer 10 additional
minutes. Serve topped with nuts.

PANACEA POTAGE
Servings: 12

1 pound dried lentils
1 pound dried split peas
½ pound dried navy beans
2–3 quarts water (as necessary)
3 leeks
1 bunch kale
1 bunch collards
1 medium eggplant, chopped
4 cups bok choy, shredded
4 carrots, ¼-inch slices
1 quart carrot juice
2 tablespoons curry powder
(optional)
2 tablespoons turmeric
4 tablespoons fresh ginger, grated
6 cloves garlic, pressed or sliced

½ cube Rapunzel Salt-Free
Bouillon
1 pound frozen blueberries
1 cup goji berries or ½ cup currants

Soak dried lentils, split peas,
and beans in water for several
hours. Drain and rinse lentils, peas,
and beans. Place in large soup kettle and add water. Simmer for 1
hour until navy beans are tender.
Add remaining ingredients, except
for blueberries and goji berries or
currants, and simmer, covered, for
another hour. Stir in remaining
ingredients just prior to serving.

Note: Be creative and make
your own vegetable potage using
vegetables and seasonings of your
choice.

NUT-CRÈME VEGETABLE SOUP
Servings: 12

4 cups natural or organic vegetable
soup (found in health food stores)
2 cups carrot juice
4 cans (15 ounces each) white
beans (navy or cannellini), salt-free
1 or 2 sheets dried sea vegetable
(kombu, hiziki, wakame, or
dulse—optional)
3 teaspoons Bragg Liquid Amino
Acids
4 cups frozen chopped broccoli

1 cup frozen chopped onion

2 cups frozen butternut squash

2 cups frozen chopped collard greens

1 cup mixed vegetables—peas, carrots, corn

½ cup raw cashews

2 teaspoons garlic powder

¼ teaspoon nutmeg

1 tablespoon Spike Salt-Free Seasoning

4 cups fresh spinach (1 bag baby spinach)

chopped walnuts (for garnish)

In a large pot, simmer first 10 ingredients for 40 minutes. Place ¼ of cooked mixture in blender with cashews, garlic powder, nutmeg, and Spike and blend until very smooth. Return mixture to pan and stir in fresh spinach. Spinach will wilt in hot soup. Serve sprinkled with chopped walnuts.

CURRIED TOMATO BISQUE
Servings: 4

1 cup finely chopped onion

2 garlic cloves, pressed

4 teaspoons curry powder

35 ounces strained tomatoes

1 cup vegetable broth

¼ cup cashew butter (preferably raw)

2 teaspoons Bragg Liquid Amino Acids

½ cup cilantro sprigs

Steam-sauté the onion, garlic, and curry powder until onions are soft, about 5 minutes. Stir in the tomatoes; cover and cook over low heat for 15 minutes. Blend soup with cashew butter and Bragg in blender until smooth. Add cilantro and pulse until finely chopped but not pureed.

SOUTHWESTERN CORN-ASPARAGUS SOUP
Servings: 6

1 large onion, chopped

1 fresh jalapeño, seeded and finely chopped

1 red bell pepper, seeded and finely chopped

4¼ cups water or vegetable stock

2 teaspoons Bragg Liquid Amino Acids

1½ pounds sweet potatoes, peeled and cut in 1-inch cubes

1 (10-ounce) package frozen organic corn

1 pound frozen cut-up asparagus

1 cup prepared mild tomato salsa

2 cloves garlic, pressed

¼ cup finely chopped cilantro

1 avocado, peeled and cubed

½ cup chopped green onions
baked corn tortilla chips

Steam-sauté onion, jalapeño, and red bell pepper in a 5- to 6-quart pot until onion is tender. Add water or stock, Bragg, and potatoes. Cover, bring to a boil, and simmer until sweet potatoes are very tender, about 12 to 14 minutes. Coarsely mash sweet potatoes in pot using potato masher. Stir in corn and asparagus and simmer for 3 minutes. Stir in salsa, garlic, and cilantro. Serve topped with avocado cubes, green onions, and a few baked tortilla chips.

QUICK GARLIC-BROCCOLI BEAN SOUP
Servings: 10

4 cups Imagine Cream of Broccoli Soup (sold in health food stores)
4 cups frozen chopped collard greens
2 cups frozen chopped broccoli
2 cups frozen Asian vegetables
2 cups frozen organic corn
2 cups carrot juice
1 can red beans, salt-free
1 can white beans, salt-free
1 can adzuki beans, salt-free

1 or 2 sheets dried sea vegetable (kombu, hiziki, wakame, or dulse—optional)
4 teaspoons garlic powder
salt-free seasoning (your choice) to taste

In a large pot, combine all ingredients, cover, and simmer for 40 minutes. Add seasonings to taste.

Note: You can use any combination of frozen vegetables you like.

PRONTO BLACK BEAN VEGETABLE SOUP
Servings: 10

4 cans (15 ounces each) black beans, salt-free if possible
4 cups natural tomato soup, low or no sodium
4 cups water
1 or 2 sheets dried sea vegetable (kombu, hiziki, wakame, or dulse—optional)
2 teaspoons Bragg Liquid Amino Acids
2 cups frozen mixed vegetables
2 cups frozen organic corn
2 cups frozen broccoli florets
4 cups carrot juice
4 teaspoons chili powder
1 teaspoon cumin
¼ cup chopped cilantro (optional)
1 cup mild tomato salsa

½ cup chopped green onions
2 avocados, chopped or mashed
½ cup raw pumpkin seeds (lightly
　roasted if you like)

Rinse beans. In a large pot, combine all ingredients except cilantro, salsa, green onions, avocado, and pumpkin seeds; bring to a boil and simmer on low for 30 minutes. Stir in salsa and heat through. Serve topped with avocado, green onions, and pumpkin seeds.

VEGETABLE ROTINI SOUP
Servings: 6

1 onion, chopped
1 cup fresh fennel bulb, chopped
2 cups sliced mushrooms
6 garlic cloves, minced
1½ tablespoons chopped fresh
　thyme
½ teaspoon dried crushed red
　pepper
4 cups water
6 cups vegetable broth
2 (24-ounce) cans chopped
　tomatoes
4 cups chopped kale (½ bunch)
2 (15-ounce) cans red kidney
　beans, rinsed and drained
7 ounces whole-grain rotini pasta
¼ cup chopped parsley

¼ cup pine nuts, lightly toasted
cold-pressed virgin olive oil

In a large saucepan, combine all ingredients except kidney beans, rotini, parsley, pine nuts, and olive oil. Simmer covered about 30 to 40 minutes until vegetables are soft. Stir in kidney beans and simmer for another 5 minutes. Add rotini and simmer until tender but still firm to the bite (about 7 to 9 minutes). To serve, sprinkle with parsley and pine nuts, and drizzle a tiny amount of olive oil on top.

SPINACH PEA SOUP
Servings: 4

10 ounces frozen green peas
1 onion, chopped
4 cloves garlic, sliced
2 teaspoons Bragg Liquid Amino
　Acids
3 pitted dates
3 cups water or vegetable stock
10 ounces baby spinach
½ cup raw cashews
4 teaspoons lemon juice
dash of Spike Salt-Free Seasoning,
　to taste
2 romaine or escarole leaves, thinly
　shredded

In a large pot, simmer peas, onion, garlic, Bragg, and dates in water or stock for about 7 minutes. Add spinach and stir until wilted, about 1 minute. Blend mixture until liquefied. Add cashews. Add additional water if necessary to reach a creamy consistency. Add lemon juice and Spike to taste. Add shredded lettuce to hot soup just prior to serving.

SPLIT PEA, LEEK, AND KALE SOUP
Servings: 8

1 pound dried split peas, rinsed
3 leeks, coarsely chopped
2 bunches kale, de-stemmed and torn in pieces
3 carrots, cut in ¼-inch rounds
6 cloves garlic, minced
1 teaspoon turmeric powder
2 teaspoons curry powder
2 teaspoons Spike Salt-Free Seasoning
4 teaspoons Bragg Liquid Amino Acids
10 cups water
6 tablespoons nutritional yeast
8 tablespoons raw sunflower seeds

In a soup kettle, combine all ingredients except yeast and sunflower seeds, cover, and simmer for 2 hours. Stir in nutritional yeast. Serve topped with sunflower seeds, one tablespoon per portion.

CURRIED LENTIL SOUP
Servings: 10

1 cup dried red lentils—do not soak
1 onion, finely chopped
6 cloves garlic, minced or pressed
2 zucchini, finely chopped
1 red bell pepper, seeded and finely chopped
2 carrots, chopped
1 or 2 sheets dried sea vegetable (kombu, hiziki, wakame, or dulse—optional)
½ teaspoon ground cumin
⅛ teaspoon ground allspice
1 teaspoon ground coriander
3 teaspoons mild curry powder
3 tablespoons grated ginger root
½ cup uncooked brown rice
4 cups carrot juice
4 cups water
4 teaspoons Bragg Liquid Amino Acids
2 sweet potatoes, cut in 1-inch cubes
2 bunches Swiss chard, chopped, stems and all
6 ounces baby spinach
½ cup currants
½ cup chopped fresh cilantro

In a soup kettle, combine all ingredients except sweet potatoes, chard, spinach, currants, and cilantro. Bring to a boil, cover, and simmer for 40 minutes. Add the potatoes and simmer for 15 minutes, then add the chard and simmer for 10 minutes. Stir in currants and spinach. When the spinach is wilted, the soup is ready. If soup is too thick, add water. Serve topped with chopped cilantro.

SAVORY VEGETABLE BEAN SOUP
Servings: 8

1 cup dried white beans, soaked in water for at least 6 hours
2 large onions
8 cups water
3 teaspoons dried mixed herbs
8 cloves garlic, sliced
6 carrots, sliced in ¼-inch rounds
½ head cabbage, shredded
1 or 2 sheets dried sea vegetable (kombu, hiziki, wakame, or dulse—optional)
3 ribs celery, coarsely chopped
4 cups kale, stems removed and coarsely chopped
3 teaspoons Bragg Liquid Amino Acids
2 teaspoons curry powder
1 cup chopped parsley
½ cup raw sunflower seeds

In pressure cooker, cook beans, onions, herbs, and garlic in 6 cups of water for 10 minutes. If using regular pot, cook covered for one hour, until beans are tender. Add vegetables, Bragg, curry powder, and remaining water to cooked beans. Simmer covered for about 20 minutes until the vegetables are tender. Serve topped with parsley and raw sunflower seeds.

BLENDED GAZPACHO SOUPS

The Spanish must have known when they created gazpacho that pureed raw vegetables are an excellent nourishment. This refreshing cold soup hails from the Andalusia region of Spain. Gazpacho means concoction, or mishmash. The gazpacho recipes are a delicious concoction of highly absorbable nutrients. Like the smoothies, gazpacho is a quick and efficient way to obtain your necessary daily nutrients. Because the nutrients are so easy for the body to absorb and assimilate, it is an excellent choice for the ill and elderly. Create your own gazpachos using any combination of non-starchy uncooked fresh produce.

You can use leftover gazpacho to make an antioxidant-rich vegetable dip or salad dressing. Add more vinegar or lime juice, raw seeds, nuts, or Tahini, and seasonings to taste.

SUMMER FRESH GAZPACHO
Servings: 2

6 large tomatoes
2 cucumbers, peeled
1 red bell pepper, seeded
½ sweet onion
1 handful fresh parsley, long stems
  removed
Bragg Liquid Amino Acids to taste
1 clove garlic, coarsely chopped
1 cup carrot juice
1 cup low-sodium tomato juice
1 avocado, mashed with lime juice
½ bunch fresh cilantro, chopped

Quarter tomatoes and remove seeds. Blend all ingredients except avocado and cilantro in blender until finely chopped. Serve topped with avocado and cilantro. Adjust seasonings to your preference.

REFRESHING WATERMELON GAZPACHO
Servings: 5

6 cups seeded watermelon
1 large ripe tomato
1 mango, peeled and seeded
1 medium cucumber, peeled and
  cut into chunks
1 red bell pepper, seeded and cut in
  pieces
2 cups white grapes
juice of 2 limes
½ cup pomegranate juice
2 cups water
¼ cup chopped fresh mint plus
  sprigs for garnish

In blender, process all ingredients except mint sprigs on medium chop. Remove half of the mixture and place in large bowl. Puree the remainder. Combine the two mixtures and serve with sprigs of mint. Adjust seasonings to your preference.

WHITE GAZPACHO
Servings: 4

1 cup blanched almonds, whole,
  slivered, or sliced
1 cup unsweetened soy milk
1 large clove garlic
½ medium onion
1 tablespoon cider vinegar or lime juice

3½ cups water
Bragg Liquid Amino Acids, to taste
1 cucumber, peeled and cut in chunks
1 cup green grapes
4 tablespoons chopped parsley

In blender, process all ingredients except parsley until pureed. Serve sprinkled with parsley.

POWER-BOOST GAZPACHO
Servings: 4

2 medium tomatoes
½ cucumber, peeled
10 grapes
½ sweet onion
1 small garlic clove
½ avocado, peeled and seeded
¼ cup raw cashews
1 tablespoon cider vinegar
1 teaspoon Bragg Liquid Amino
   Acids
3 handfuls baby spinach

In blender, blend all ingredients until smooth. Adjust seasonings to your preference.

HEARTY GAZPACHO
Servings: 2

1 small cucumber
½ red bell pepper, seeded

1 small carrot
1 crown broccoli
2 medium tomatoes
½ medium onion
½ cup cooked or canned white
   beans (navy or Great Northern),
   rinsed
1 clove garlic
2 cups low-sodium tomato juice
Bragg Liquid Amino Acids, to taste
1 tablespoon nutritional yeast

Cut vegetables in chunks, combine all ingredients in a blender, and puree. Adjust seasonings to your taste.

GREEN GAZPACHO
Servings: 4

1 large cucumber, peeled and cut
   into chunks
1 green bell pepper, seeded and cut
   into pieces
1 stalk celery, cut into pieces
juice of 1 lime
1 cup white grapes
2 tablespoons chopped green onion
   or chives
2 cups low-sodium tomato juice
Bragg Liquid Amino Acids, to taste
1 tablespoon nutritional yeast
2 cups coarsely chopped chard

In food processor or blender, puree all ingredients. Adjust tartness and seasonings to your preference.

STEWS

QUICK VEGETABLE-BEAN CHILI
Servings: 8

10 ounces frozen onions
3 cups finely chopped frozen
    broccoli
3 cups finely chopped frozen
cauliflower
3 cloves garlic, pressed or minced
1 can pinto beans, salt-free
1 can black beans, salt-free
1 can red beans, salt-free
2 (28-ounce) cans diced tomatoes,
    no salt added
1 small can chopped mild green
    chili
3 tablespoons mild chili powder, or
    more to taste
1 teaspoon cumin
2½ cups fresh or frozen organic
    corn
2 large zucchinis, finely chopped
2 teaspoons Bragg Liquid Amino
    Acids
4 tablespoons nutritional yeast
1½ cups tomato salsa
2 avocados, mashed

In large pot, combine all ingredients except yeast, salsa, and avocado; cover and simmer over low heat for 2 hours. Stir in nutritional yeast, and serve topped with salsa and avocado.

AFRICAN GROUND-NUT
VEGETABLE STEW
Servings: 6

2 cups chopped frozen onions
2 cups chopped carrots
1 pound mushrooms (any kind),
    sliced
1 pound chopped frozen collard
    greens (or any other chopped
    greens)
3 cups chopped frozen broccoli
1 pound frozen okra
1 (24-ounce) can chopped
    tomatoes (lowest sodium)
3 teaspoons Bragg Liquid Amino
    Acids
8 cloves garlic, pressed or minced
2 cups water
1¼ teaspoons ground ginger
1 teaspoon ground cumin
1 tablespoon chili powder
¾ teaspoon ground coriander
4 teaspoons curry powder
1 tablespoon ground cinnamon
⅔ cup unsalted peanut butter or
    raw almond butter

4 cups fresh or frozen carrot juice,
or just water

½ tablespoon currants or raisins
(more if you like)

2 (15-ounce) cans garbanzo beans,
salt-free

3 cups fresh fruit (apple, pear,
peach), coarsely chopped

Put vegetables, tomatoes, Bragg,
garlic, and water in soup kettle and
bring to a simmer. In a separate
bowl, whisk nut butter with carrot
juice until blended. Add to soup
kettle and simmer covered for 30
to 45 minutes. Add currants and
garbanzos and simmer covered for
another 10 minutes. Serve topped
with fresh fruit.

TOFU-VEGETABLE CHILI
Servings: 16

2 pounds extra firm tofu, frozen
and thawed

6 tablespoons mild chili powder—
use less if you prefer

1 large green bell pepper, seeded
and coarsely chopped

1 large red bell pepper, seeded and
coarsely chopped

2 medium onions, coarsely
chopped

1 pound chopped frozen broccoli

2 cups frozen organic corn

1 pound chopped frozen collard
greens

8 cloves garlic, minced or pressed

2 (28-ounce) plus 1 (15-ounce)
cans stewed or chopped tomatoes

1 (8-ounce) can chopped green
chilis

1 (15-ounce) can cooked kidney
beans, no salt added or drain and
rinse well

1 (15-ounce) can cooked pinto
beans, no salt added or drain and
rinse well

1 (15-ounce) can cooked black
beans, no salt added or drain and
rinse well

(freshly cooked tomatoes and
beans can replace the canned
variety—use same quantities)

Squeeze excess water out of
thawed tofu and crumble. Coat
bottom of a 1-gallon or larger soup
pot with olive oil, and brown
crumbled tofu quickly with chili
powder. Add remaining ingredients
and simmer on low heat for 1½ to
2 hours.

SPECIAL CHILI BEANS
Servings: 6

1 (15-ounce) can pinto beans, salt-
free or drained and rinsed

1 (15-ounce) can black beans, salt-free or drained and rinsed

1 (15-ounce) can red beans, salt-free or drained and rinsed

10 ounces frozen onions

1 pound chopped frozen broccoli

3 cloves garlic, minced

1 (28-ounce) can diced tomatoes, no salt added

1 small can chopped mild green chili

4 tablespoons mild chili powder (or more to taste)

2 teaspoons cumin

½ cup natural ketchup

2 large zucchini, diced

3 teaspoons Bragg Liquid Amino Acids

1 cup currants

4 tablespoons raw almond butter

In a soup kettle, combine all ingredients except currants and almond butter, and simmer, covered, for 45 minutes. Stir in currants and almond butter.

Note: Good kid dish.

MAIN DISHES

ASIAN-MEXICAN FUSION STIR-FRY
Servings: 4

2 cups small broccoli florets

2 cups small or sliced mushrooms

½ cup sugar snap peas or snow peas, stringed

1 small onion, cut in wedges and separated into 1-inch strips

2 medium red bell peppers, seeded and cut in 1-inch squares

1 cup bok choy, cut in bite-sized pieces

1 medium carrot, cut diagonally into ⅓-inch slices

3 cans red beans

8 ounces fresh spinach

¼ cup raw cashews (optional)

2 cups finely shredded Chinese cabbage

2 cups cooked brown rice

2 tablespoons unhulled sesame seeds, lightly toasted in dry skillet until lightly browned and popping

Sauce

3 tablespoons of store-bought 100% fruit peach or apricot spread

2 cups carrot juice

1 tablespoon grated ginger root

2 cloves garlic, pressed or minced

3 teaspoons Bragg Liquid Amino Acids

2 teaspoons cornstarch or 3 teaspoons arrowroot powder

3 tablespoons unsalted peanut butter or unsalted raw almond butter

pepper flakes to taste

For the sauce, combine ingredients in blender; blend until smooth and set aside.

Steam-sauté first seven stir-fry ingredients over medium-high heat, covered but tossing often, cooking vegetables about 5 minutes or so. Add more water as necessary to keep from scorching. Add sauce and beans; simmer covered and stirring often until veggies are just tender. Add more water if needed. Add spinach, toss until wilted. Mix cashews in and serve over microwave-warmed shredded Chinese cabbage and a small portion of brown rice. Top with sesame seeds.

SWEET POTATO–VEGETABLE PIE
Servings: 8

8 sweet potatoes
3 cups chopped fresh or frozen broccoli
2 cups chopped frozen collard greens
2 cups fresh or frozen cauliflower
2 cups chopped fresh or frozen onions
½ pound white mushrooms, sliced
½ pound shiitake mushrooms, sliced
6 cloves garlic, pressed

1 red bell pepper, seeded and cut into 1-inch squares
2½ cups water
¼ cube Rapunzel Salt-Free Vegan vegetable bouillon (found in health food stores)
3 teaspoons mild chili powder
3 tablespoons tomato paste
2 teaspoons Bragg Liquid Amino Acids
2 tablespoons raw nut butter (any kind)
3 cups cooked or canned red beans
½ cup chopped pecans

Use leftover mashed sweet potatoes, or in a 375-degree oven prick and bake sweet potatoes until soft, about 40 minutes to an hour. When potatoes are tender, peel, put in a bowl, and mash.

In a large pot, combine broccoli, collard greens, cauliflower, onions, mushrooms, and bell pepper in water and simmer covered for 15 minutes. Add bouillon, chili powder, tomato paste, and Bragg and cook until almost tender (about 10 minutes). Mix in nut butter and beans and spread the mixture in a baking dish. Spread sweet potatoes over the top and sprinkle with a little additional chili powder and chopped pecans. Bake 20 to 30 minutes until hot and

Food for Life

Basic Cooked Black Beans
with Avocado, Tomatoes,
Cilantro, and Lime

Savory Vegetable-
Bean Soup

Carol Crosthwait 2007

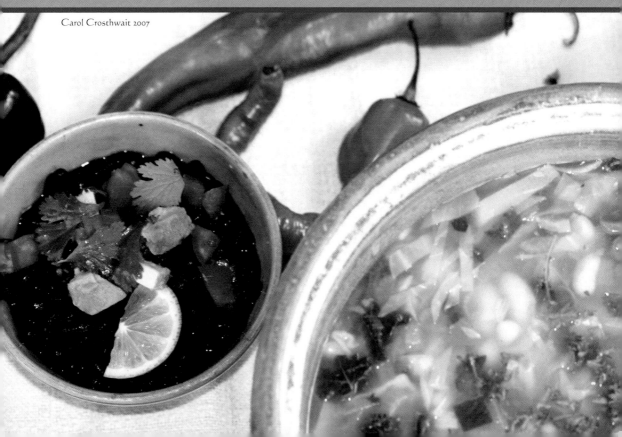

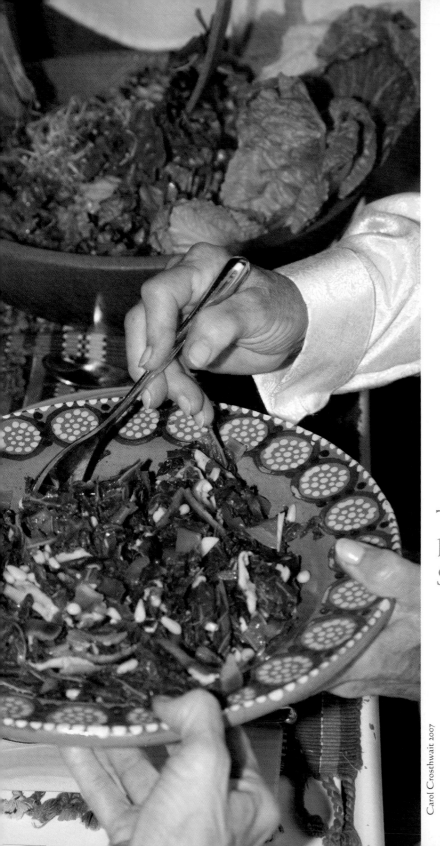

Tuscan
Kale-Mushroom
Sauté

Carol Crosthwait 2007

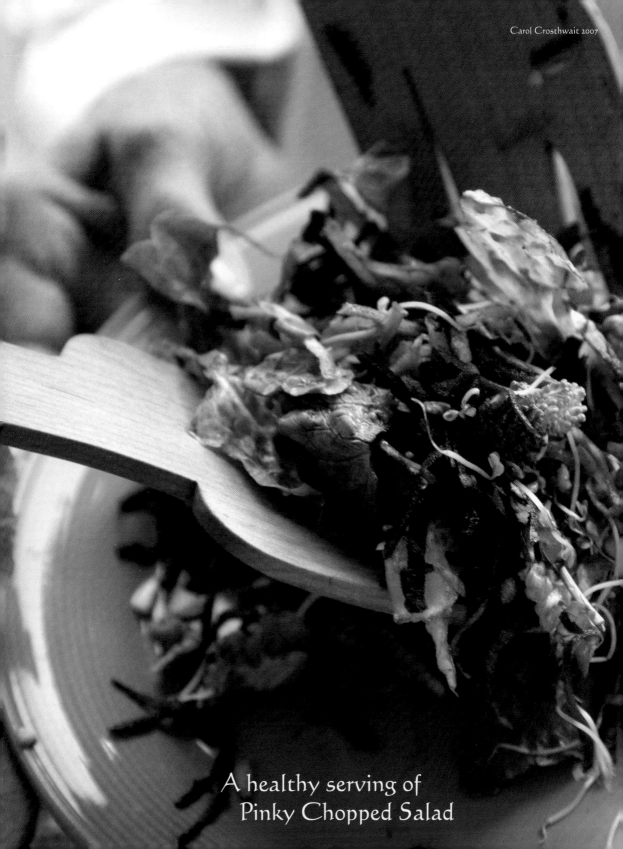

Carol Crosthwait 2007

A healthy serving of
Pinky Chopped Salad

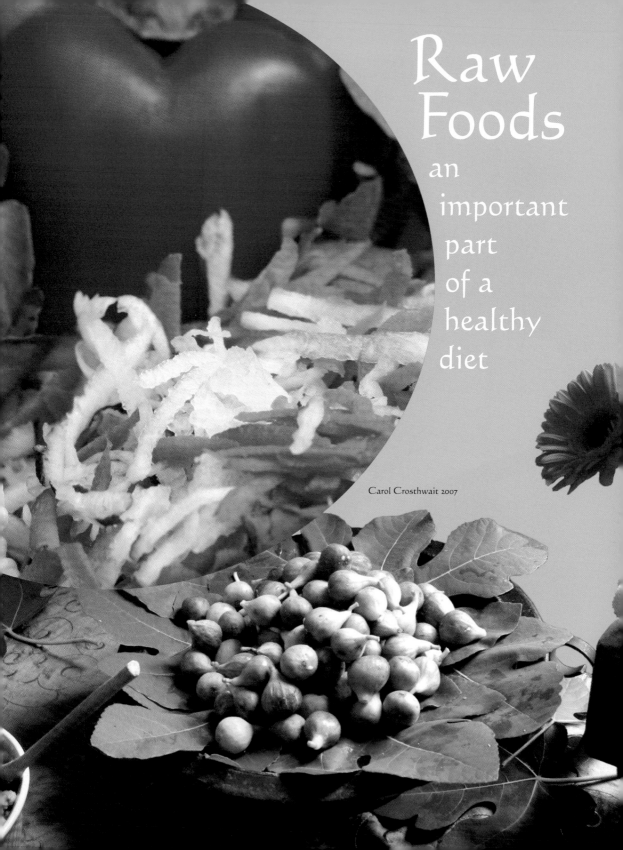

Raw Foods

an important part of a healthy diet

Carol Crosthwait 2007

Fresh from the Garden

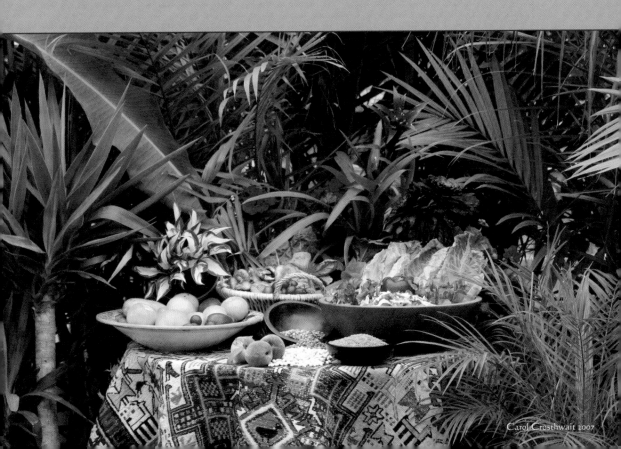

Carol Crosthwait 2007

Sake Steamed Wild Salmon with Orange-Ginger Sauce on a Bed of Steamed Bok Choy

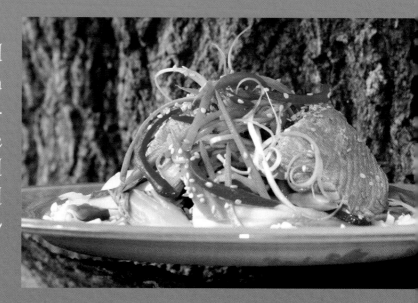

All photos by Carol Crosthwait 2007

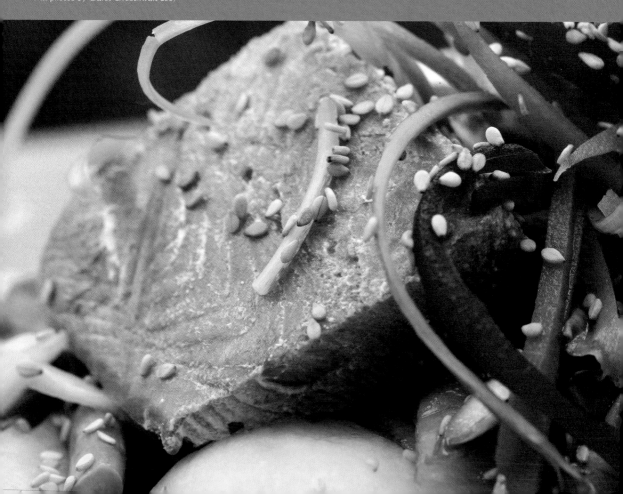

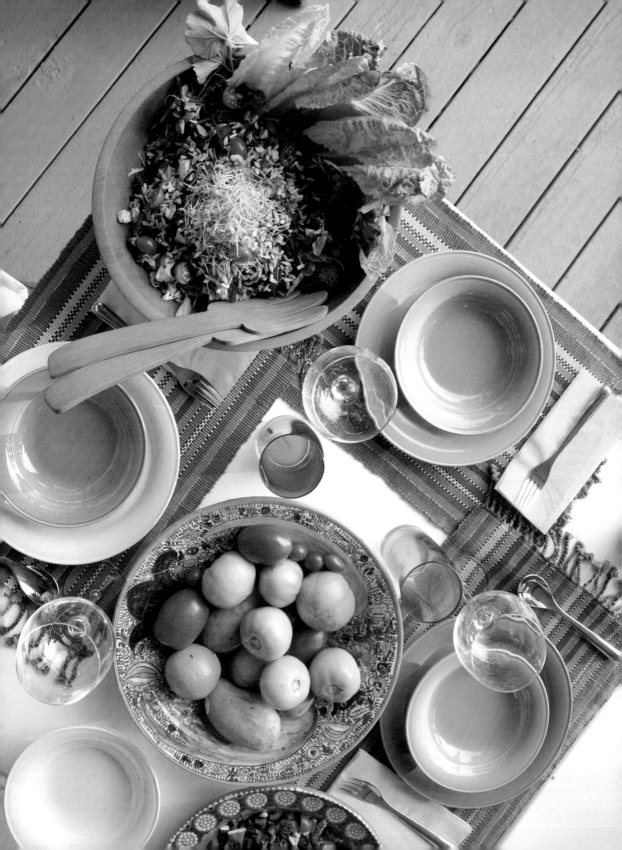

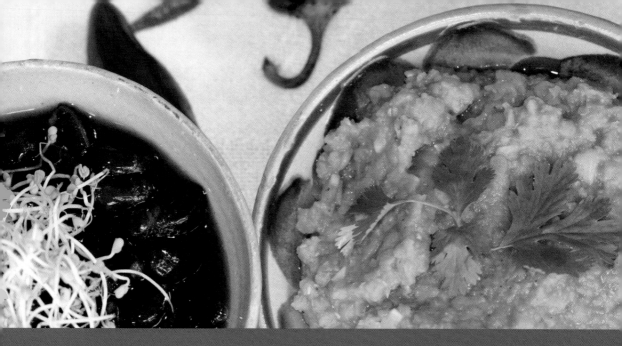

Basic Cooked Red Beans   Basic Red Lentils

Asian-Style Chopped Salad • Robin's Favorite Chopped
Salad • Vibrant Fruit Salad with Cherry-Berry Dressing

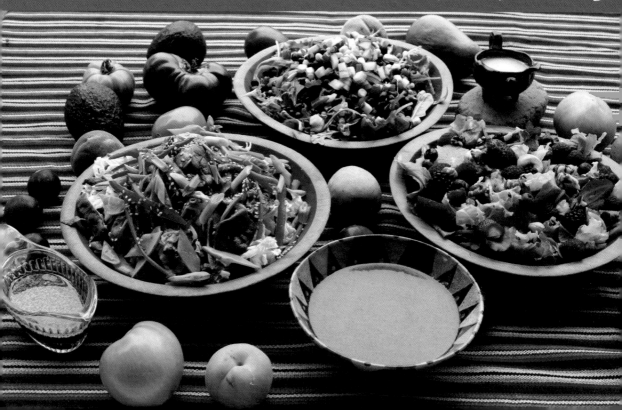

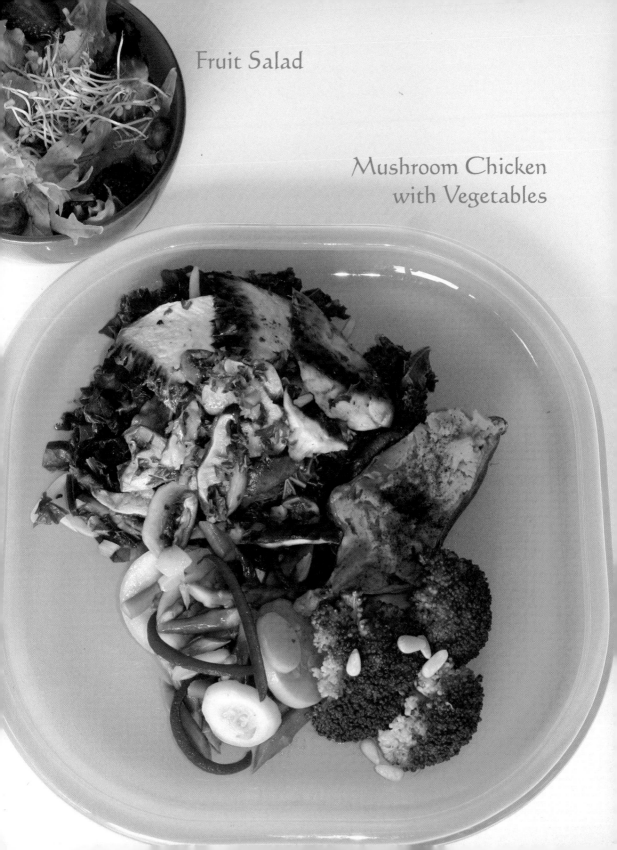

Fruit Salad

Mushroom Chicken
with Vegetables

Curried Red Lentils

Pomegranate Poached
    Pears with Berry-Berry Sauce

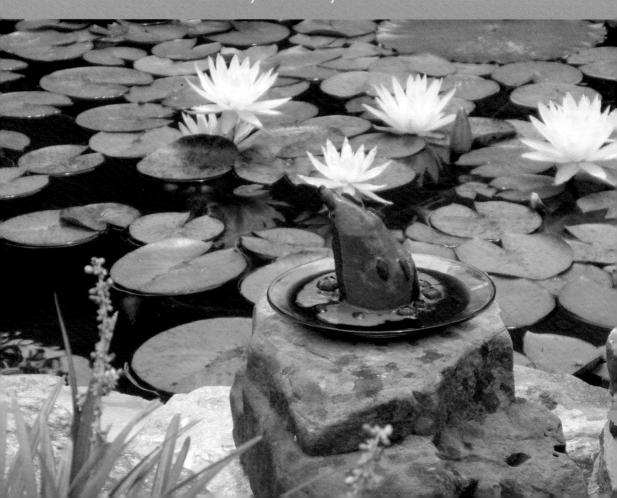

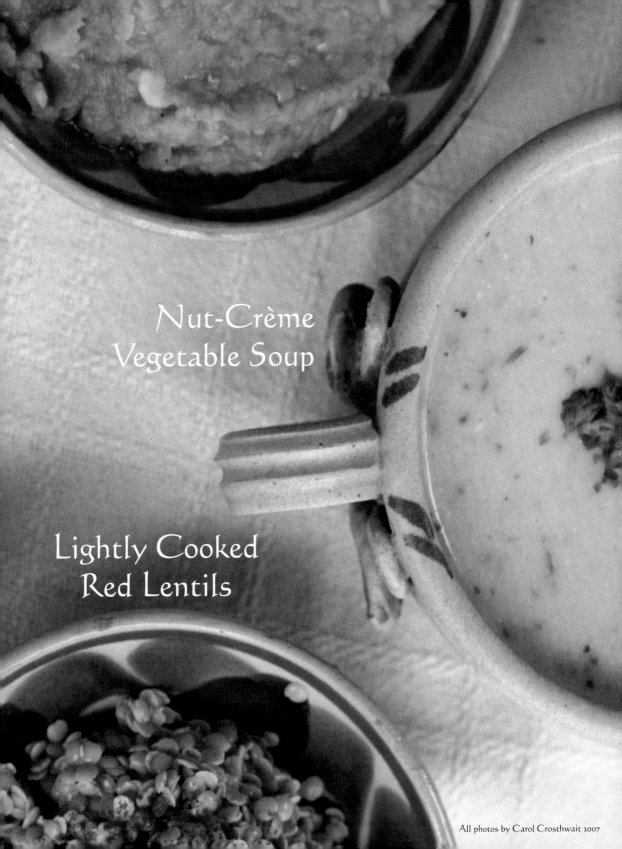

Nut-Crème
Vegetable Soup

Lightly Cooked
Red Lentils

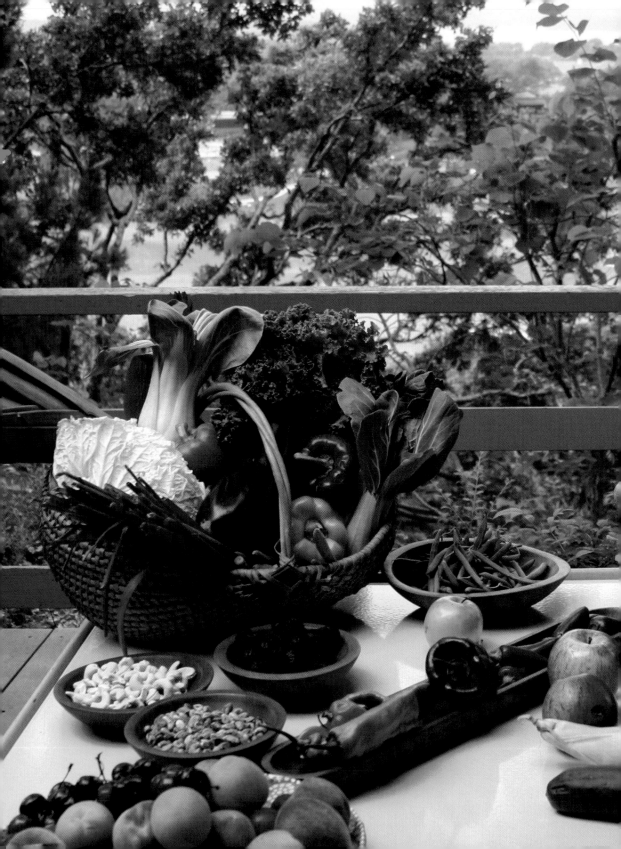

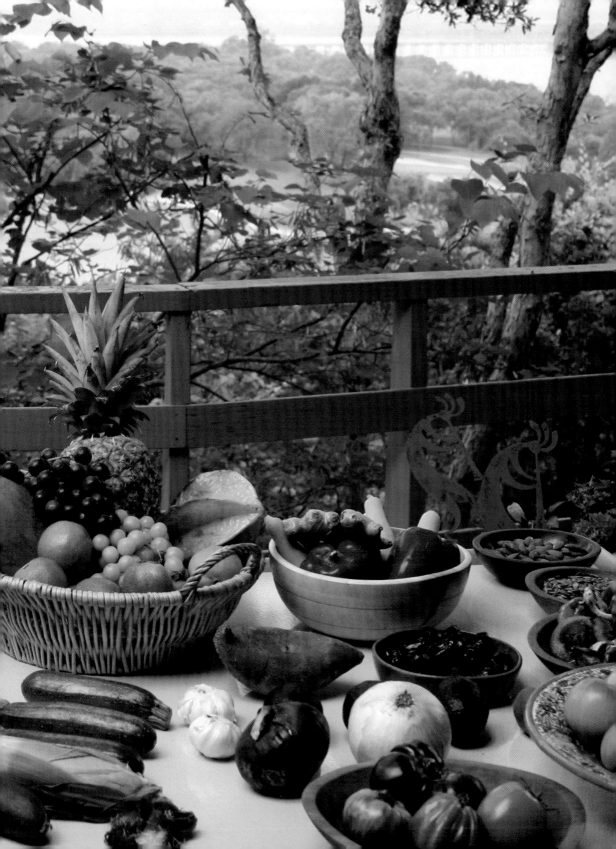

Vibrant Asparagus, Bean,
and Mushroom Salad

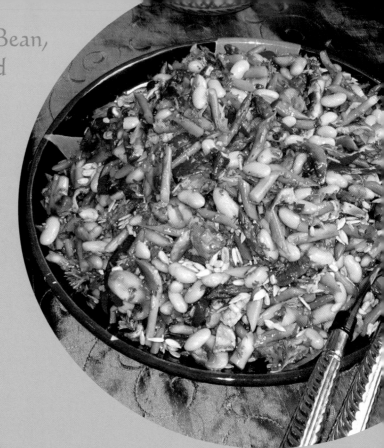

Basic Grilled Salmon

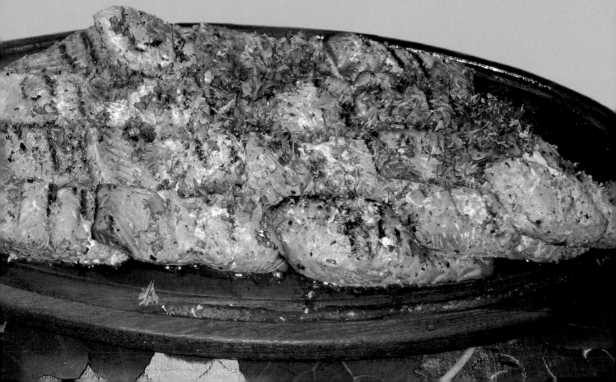

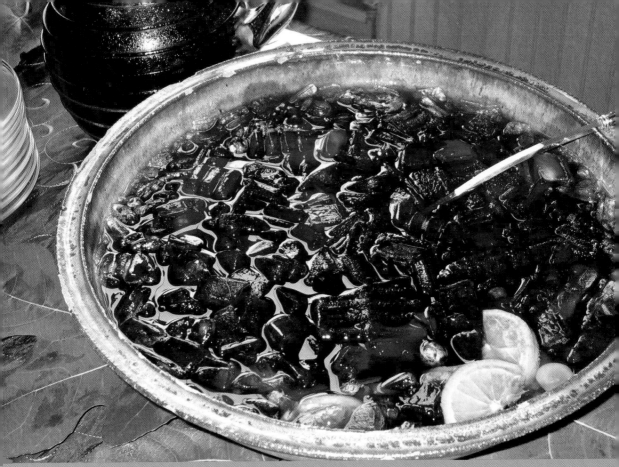

Refreshing Antioxidant Tea Punch with Fruit

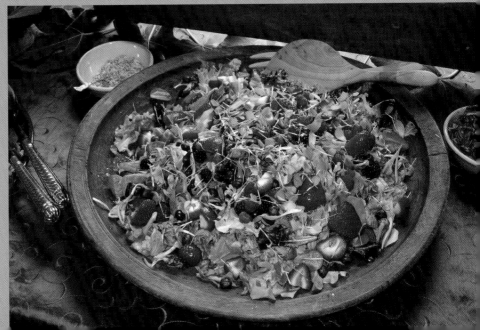

Confetti
Salad

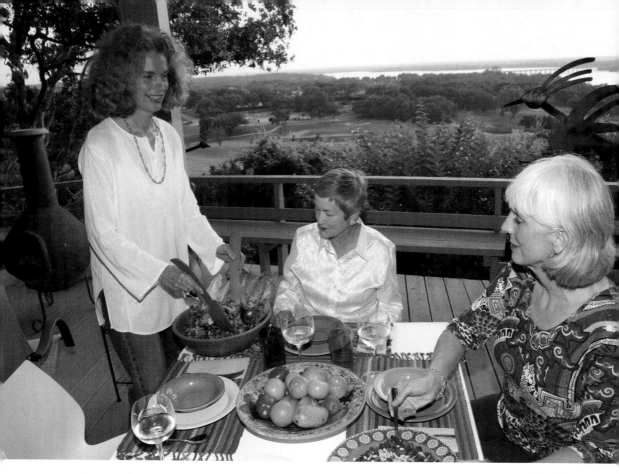

Carol Crosthwait 200

A healthy, antioxidant-rich
meal prepared by Chef Robin

pecans are light brown, about 20 minutes if warm, and about 30 minutes if coming from refrigerator.

Note: This dish can be prepared ahead and frozen, baked or unbaked.

INDIAN VEGETABLE CURRY
Servings: 6

2 cups red lentils

3 cups water

3 cups carrot juice

1 onion, chopped

1 green bell pepper, seeded and chopped

8 garlic cloves, pressed or minced

2 tablespoons curry powder

2 teaspoons garam masala (dried, ground spice mix found in Indian or health food stores)

1 cinnamon stick

1½ teaspoons chili powder

2 cups chopped Italian plum tomatoes, drained

2 cups water

2 teaspoons Bragg Liquid Amino Acids

4 carrots, halved lengthwise and cut into ½-inch pieces

2 sweet potatoes, peeled and cubed

1 cauliflower, trimmed and cut into small florets

2 cups halved Brussels sprouts

2 (15-ounce) cans garbanzo beans, rinsed and drained

3 tablespoons currants

4 cups cooked quinoa or brown rice

¼ cup chopped fresh cilantro

½ cup raw cashew pieces

In large pot, combine the first 10 ingredients. Cover and simmer for about 20 minutes, until lentils are soft. Add the next 7 ingredients and simmer for 15 to 20 minutes until vegetables are tender. Stir in garbanzo beans and currants, and cook for 5 minutes longer. Remove cinnamon stick, and serve with quinoa or brown rice. Sprinkle with cilantro and cashew pieces.

VEGGIE WRAPS
Servings: 4

1 cup cooked or canned lentils or beans

½ cup chopped celery

1 orange, peeled, sectioned, and seeded

½ teaspoon garlic, pressed or minced

½ tablespoon balsamic vinegar

3 teaspoons cold-pressed virgin olive oil

1 tablespoon dried currants

¼ cup chopped red bell pepper (seeds removed)

1 tablespoon chopped parsley

1 tablespoon chopped mint
1 teaspoon Bragg Liquid Amino
   Acids
1 tablespoon nutritional yeast
¼ cup coarsely chopped walnuts
12 large leaf lettuce leaves

Combine all ingredients except for lettuce leaves. Spread mixture on each lettuce leaf and roll.

TUSCAN-BAKED SQUASH WITH TOMATO-VEGETABLE-BEAN SAUCE
Servings: 4–6

1 large butternut or spaghetti
   squash
4 cloves garlic, pressed
1 teaspoon ground cinnamon
1 (28-ounce) can low-sodium
   chopped tomatoes
4 cups kale, de-stemmed and torn
   in bite-sized pieces (can substitute frozen kale or greens)
1 onion, chopped
1 pound fresh mushrooms (any
   kind—an assortment is ideal),
   sliced
1 ounce dried porcini mushrooms,
   reconstituted and coarsely
   chopped (optional, but adds flavor)
8 cloves garlic, minced
½ cup raisins

2 teaspoons Bragg Liquid Amino
   Acids
3 (15-ounce) cans cannellini or
   navy beans, salt-free
6 Roma tomatoes, chopped
2 bags (5 to 7 ounces) organic baby
   spinach
1 bunch basil (about ½ cup
   chopped), plus 3 whole sprigs
3 tablespoons pine nuts

Preheat oven to 350 degrees. Microwave butternut squash for 8 minutes to soften, then cut in half lengthwise. Scrape out seeds. Spread the 4 cloves of pressed garlic on the inside of each half and place 1½ sprigs of basil in each cavity. Sprinkle the interiors with cinnamon. Put the two halves back together and place on a baking sheet. Bake for 1 hour or until tender. In large saucepan, simmer canned tomatoes, kale, onion, mushrooms, minced garlic, raisins, Bragg, and beans for 20 minutes. Add fresh tomatoes, spinach, and chopped basil and continue to simmer until spinach wilts. Remove baked squash, separate halves, and cut in large chunks. If you use spaghetti squash, rough it up with the prongs of a fork before serving. Serve squash topped with sauce and pine nuts.

EASY STUFFED EGGPLANT OR CABBAGE ROLLS
Servings: 6

2 large eggplants, cut in ½-inch thick lengthwise slices
2 medium red bell peppers, seeded and coarsely chopped into ¼-inch pieces
½ cup chopped celery
1 cup coarsely chopped carrots
1 medium onion or 3 leeks, coarsely chopped
½ pound fresh shiitake or button mushrooms, sliced
4 cloves garlic, chopped
8 ounces fresh spinach, shredded
1 teaspoon Bragg Liquid Amino Acids
2 cups tomato pasta sauce (lowest sodium you can find)
6 ounces mozzarella cheese substitute, shredded
1 (15-ounce) can red beans, rinsed and drained
¼ cup raw pine nuts

Lightly oil a nonstick baking ban. Place eggplant in a single layer. Bake at 350 degrees about 20 minutes or until the eggplant is flexible enough to roll easily.

Water-sauté the bell pepper, celery, carrots, onion, mushrooms, and garlic until just tender. Add spinach and Bragg. Take off heat and place in mixing bowl. Toss in 2 to 3 tablespoons of tomato sauce, shredded soy cheese, beans, and pine nuts. In a baking pan, spread about ¼ cup tomato sauce. Put some of mixture on each eggplant slice, roll, and place in baking pan on top of sauce. Pour remaining tomato sauce over eggplant rolls. Bake in a 350-degree oven until hot throughout.

Note: You can also make stuffed cabbage rolls with this stuffing. Blanch a whole head of cabbage in boiling water. Remove individual leaves as they become soft and pliable, and return cabbage to water to remove next leaf. Do this until you have 12 leaves, or as many as needed. Place stuffing on leaves and roll from base, tucking leaves in on the sides. Arrange and bake according to eggplant instructions.

SOUTHWESTERN AVOCADO BEAN WRAP
Servings: 4

1 cup black beans, cooked or canned
1 tomato, chopped
1 avocado, cubed
¼ cup fresh or frozen organic corn, uncooked

¼ cup chopped green onions

½ cup cucumber, small cubes

½ teaspoon garlic, minced or pressed

1 teaspoon Bragg Liquid Amino Acids

3 teaspoons lime juice

3 teaspoons cold-pressed virgin olive oil

1 tablespoon chopped cilantro

1 teaspoon minced jalapeño

4 Ezekiel Sprouted Grain Tortillas

4 lettuce leaves

Combine all ingredients except tortillas and lettuce. Warm tortillas. Lay lettuce leaf on tortilla. Spread filling and roll.

VEGETABLE PIZZA
Servings: 2

2 cups broccoli florets

1 large red bell pepper, seeded and sliced 1 inch thick

1 large Portobello mushroom, sliced ½ inch thick

1 teaspoon garlic powder

½ teaspoon Bragg Liquid Amino Acids

1 tablespoon balsamic vinegar

1 teaspoon salt-free dry seasoning mix

½ cup low-salt pasta sauce

2 Ezekiel Sprouted Grain Tortillas

4 ounces soy or rice cheese substitute, grated

5 ounces fresh spinach or 1 bag organic baby spinach, wilted in steamer or microwave

Preheat oven to 350 degrees. In a large bowl, toss broccoli, bell peppers, and mushrooms with garlic, Bragg, vinegar, and seasoning mix. Roast vegetables on a lightly oiled cookie sheet, turning occasionally and mounding to keep from drying out, for 30 minutes. Remove vegetables when done and preheat oven to 450 degrees. Spread a thin layer of pasta sauce on tortilla, sprinkle cheese, and distribute roasted vegetables and spinach. Bake on a cookie sheet for approximately 7 minutes or until cheese is melted and tortilla browns around edges.

Note: Also a great way to use leftover vegetables. Some people like to add sliced fruit to the vegetable mix.

ANTIOXIDANT LASAGNA
Servings: 8

2 large eggplants, sliced ½ inch crosswise

1 pound fresh mushrooms, sliced

2 teaspoons Spike or Mrs. Dash
  salt-free seasoning
3 cups pasta sauce (look for lowest
  in sodium)
4 medium zucchini, grated
2 carrots, grated
2 crowns broccoli, chopped, or ½
  package shredded broccoli salad
  mix (fresh produce department)
1 red pepper, chopped
1 onion, chopped
8 cloves garlic, minced or chopped
3 whole-grain lasagna leaves,
  uncooked
1 (7-ounce) bag organic baby
  spinach
1 bunch fresh basil, shredded

Tofu Ricotta

1½ pounds extra firm tofu, squeeze
  water and crumble
2 tablespoons dried Italian herbs
7 ounces soy mozzarella cheese,
  grated
¼ cup soy parmesan (optional)

Preheat oven to 350 degrees.
Bake eggplant slices in a lightly
oiled baking pan for 15 minutes
until flexible but not completely
cooked.

Combine tofu ricotta ingredients and set aside.

Steam-sauté mushrooms and
Spike or Mrs. Dash seasoning until
liquid is cooked off.

In a bowl, combine vegetables
(not the spinach) and garlic.

To assemble: Spread a layer of
pasta sauce on bottom of a very
large baking dish. Layer, pressing
with hands as you go, half of the
eggplant slices, half of the raw
spinach leaves, one layer lasagna
sheets, pasta sauce, vegetables,
remaining eggplant and spinach,
tofu ricotta, and shredded basil,
and spread with pasta sauce. Cover
with foil and bake 1½ hours or
until very hot and bubbly. Garnish
with more shredded fresh basil if
you like.

ANTIOXIDANT THAI VEGETABLE CURRY
Servings: 8

4 cups carrot juice
½ cup unsweetened coconut milk
2 tablespoons apricot 100% fruit
  spread
6 cloves garlic, finely chopped
1-inch piece fresh ginger root
6 sprigs fresh mint leaves
1 bunch fresh basil leaves
½ bunch fresh cilantro leaves
3 tablespoons unsalted peanut, raw
  cashew, or raw almond butter
1 teaspoon Bragg Liquid Amino
  Acids

½ teaspoon curry powder (add Thai curry paste for a spicier sauce to taste)

1 red bell pepper, seeded and thinly sliced

1 large eggplant, cut in 1-inch cubes

2 cups green beans, cut in 2-inch lengths

3 cups sliced shiitake and button mushrooms

1 can bamboo shoots, sliced

2 pounds tofu cut in ¼-inch thick slices

1 bunch fresh spinach, torn in pieces

4 cups cooked Wehani or brown rice

In blender, combine carrot juice, coconut milk, fruit spread, garlic, ginger, mint, basil, cilantro, nut butter, Bragg, and curry powder. (Save some whole fresh herb sprigs for garnish and seasoning.) Finely chop and blend. Place all ingredients, except rice and garnish herbs, in wok or large skillet. Bring to a boil and simmer covered, stirring occasionally, until all vegetables are tender. Add spinach right before serving. Serve on top of cooked rice, topped with sprigs of fresh herbs.

STUFFED BELL PEPPERS
Servings: 6

8 small red peppers (use different colors for vibrancy), slice off tops and gently remove seeds to make cups for filling—save the tops

½ cup quinoa

1 small red pepper, chopped

½ pound mushrooms, chopped

3 whole green onions, chopped

2 stalks celery, chopped

1 stalk broccoli, chopped in small pieces

4 cloves garlic, minced or pressed

½ cup raisins

½ bunch parsley, chopped

2 ounces mozzarella cheese substitute (I like Soya Kaas)

2 cups cooked legumes or canned no- or low-salt, rinsed and drained

½ cup coarsely chopped walnuts

2 teaspoons Bragg Liquid Amino Acids

2 cups low sodium pasta sauce

Preheat the oven to 350 degrees. On baking sheet, bake peppers and tops about 15 minutes or until slightly flexible.

Cook quinoa (½ cup quinoa to 1 cup water): Bring to a boil; turn down to low and simmer covered for 15 minutes. Take off heat and let it sit covered for 10 minutes.

Water-sauté chopped vegetables (not the parsley) and garlic until tender and water has cooked off. In large bowl, mix cooked quinoa, nuts, soy cheese, and half the parsley with all sautéed ingredients and season with Bragg and any herbs and/or no-salt seasoning you like. Fill peppers with filling, spoon pasta sauce over filling, put the pepper lid on top, and place each pepper in a baking dish. Spoon some pasta sauce over the peppers. Bake for 20 to 30 minutes until hot. Delicious served on a bed of salad greens lightly tossed with balsamic vinegar. Garnish vegetables with remaining chopped parsley.

Note: The filling is great for stuffed portobello mushrooms or other vegetables.

MAIN DISHES
(Animal Products)
FISH

BASIC GRILLED SALMON
Servings: 4

1¼ pounds wild salmon, cut into
    4-ounce portions
juice of 2 lemons

4 cloves garlic, pressed
Spike Salt-Free Seasoning

Place fish on plate and marinate in lemon juice, Spike, and garlic in the refrigerator for 30 minutes.

Heat grill to high with lid closed for 10 minutes until very hot. Place salmon skin-side down on grill. Just lightly brown salmon on each side (about 7 minutes or until center is done, silky not dry) and remove from grill. Remove skin.

Oven broiler method: You can also broil the salmon in the oven. Preheat broiler and broil fish on one side until browned, flip, and broil the other side.

Pan grill method: Spray skillet with olive oil. Heat skillet over high heat until hot. Cook salmon over medium-high heat about 7 minutes, or until browned, and do the same on the other side about 3 to 7 minutes until meat is just cooked through. Some people like the meat slightly rare. You can check it by pulling it apart in the middle with a fork. It should be done through but silky in the center. Do not overcook.

Serve with lemon slices or salsa.

PECAN-ENCRUSTED WILD SALMON
Servings: 4

1 pound wild salmon, cut into 4-
    ounce portions, skin removed
juice of 2 lemons
5 cloves garlic, pressed
Spike Salt-Free Seasoning
⅔ cup chopped raw pecans
2 teaspoons Worcestershire sauce
1 teaspoon chili powder
1 teaspoon cold-pressed olive oil

Preheat oven to 450 degrees.
Marinate the salmon with lemon
juice, two-thirds of the garlic, and a
generous portion of Spike sprinkled on top. Place in refrigerator
while preparing other ingredients.

Mix chopped pecans,
Worcestershire sauce, chili powder,
remainder of garlic, and olive oil.
Spread nut mixture over top of fish
and gently pack down. Bake for 8
to 10 minutes until silky, not dry,
in center. Bake approximately 10
minutes per inch thickness of flesh.

SAKE STEAMED WILD SALMON WITH ORANGE GINGER SAUCE
Servings: 4

2 carrots
7 green onions, with green tops
1 red bell pepper, seeded
2 cups coarsely shredded bok choy
2 cups broccoli florets
½ pound shiitake mushrooms,
    stems removed and sliced
10 ounces baby spinach
1 pound wild salmon, skin removed
    and divided into 4 (4-ounce)
    portions
2 cups sake (Japanese rice wine)
1 cup water
4 slices fresh ginger
2 cups cooked brown rice
¼ cup sesame seeds

Sauce

1 tablespoon minced fresh ginger
3 tablespoons seasoned rice wine
    (sake)
4 teaspoons Bragg Liquid Amino
    Acids
1 tablespoon cashew butter
1 cup orange juice

In a small bowl, whisk the sauce
ingredients and set aside.

Prepare garnish by thinly slicing
1 carrot, making very thin julienne
strips. Thinly slice 2 green onions
lengthwise. Thinly slice a small
amount of red bell pepper. Place all
strips in ice water. The onions will
curl nicely. This makes a beautiful
wispy garnish.

Cut remaining red bell pepper
in bite-sized pieces. Cut 3 green

onions in 1-inch pieces on the diagonal. Steam-sauté these vegetables with bok choy, broccoli, and mushrooms until tender, about 8 to 10 minutes; add spinach and wilt for 1 minute. Set aside to be warmed before serving.

Place fish in covered skillet with sake, water, several slices of ginger, 2 whole green onions, and 1 whole carrot. Bring to a boil and simmer for 10 minutes per 1-inch thickness of fish. Do not overcook. The fish should be silky inside, not dry.

Place rice on plate, top with vegetables, then steamed fish. Pour sauce over fish, vegetables, and rice. Top with garnish and sprinkle with sesame seeds.

Note: An elegant dinner party dish.

TOMATO-TOPPED WILD SALMON ON ASPARAGUS AND SPINACH
Servings: 4

1¼ pounds wild salmon, skinned
   and cut into 4-ounce portions
juice of 2 lemons
4 cloves garlic, pressed
Spike Salt-Free Seasoning
1½ pounds fresh asparagus
2 teaspoons cold-pressed olive oil

4 ½-inch slices of tomato
1 bunch (16 ounces) fresh spinach

Marinate the salmon with lemon juice, two-thirds of the garlic, and a generous portion of Spike sprinkled on top. Place in refrigerator while preparing other ingredients.

Thinly shred spinach. Hold an asparagus spear at both ends and bend; it will break where the woody ends begin. Use that spear as a guide to cut the others. Toss asparagus in olive oil and remaining pressed garlic.

Heat grill on high with lid closed for 10 minutes until very hot. Grill fish, asparagus, and tomatoes with lid closed on high for about 3 minutes. Turn asparagus and close the lid for another 2 or 3 minutes. Do not overcook tomatoes, just lightly brown on each side and remove. Remove asparagus and flip salmon; grill for another 5 minutes or until silky in the center.

Or use broiler on high heat. Cook on one side for approximately 5 minutes. Turn fish; remove skin if it was not previously removed (removes easily when cooked). Grill uncovered on medium high for at least another 3 to 7 minutes (depending on thickness) or until cooked through. Should be silky in the center.

Make a bed of shredded spinach on dinner plate and place generous portion of asparagus on spinach. Top salmon with grilled tomato and serve.

Note: Use remaining 4 ounces grilled salmon for next day's Salmon Veggie Wrap, Wild Salmon Chowder, or Wild Salmon Salad Niçoise.

WILD SALMON CHOWDER
Servings: 6

4 medium sweet potatoes, peeled and cubed
2 leeks, chopped
½ cup chopped carrots
1 cup chopped celery
⅔ cup chopped bell pepper (red, green, and yellow), seeds removed
¼ cup white wine
5 cups water
2 bay leaves
3 teaspoons Bragg Liquid Amino Acids
8 ounces salmon, cooked, canned, or raw, cut into bite-sized pieces (if canned, rinse and remove skin)
1 cup frozen peas
1 cup frozen organic corn

1 cup unsweetened soy milk
½ cup chopped parsley

In a large pot, combine potatoes, leeks, carrots, celery, bell pepper, white wine, water, Bragg, and bay leaves and simmer covered until vegetables and potatoes are tender, for about 15 to 20 minutes. Discard bay leaf. With slotted spoon, reserve about 1 cup of cooked vegetables. Blend remaining cooked ingredients and broth in blender to liquefy. Return thickened potato-vegetable stock to saucepan and add reserved cooked vegetables, salmon, peas, and corn. Simmer for 7 minutes until salmon is cooked. Add soy milk and heat through. Serve garnished with chopped parsley.

BAKED WILD SNAPPER FLORENTINE WITH ARTICHOKES AND TOMATOES
Servings: 4

1 small onion, quartered and thinly sliced
4 cloves garlic, chopped
⅓ cup dry white wine
1 (9-ounce) package frozen artichoke hearts, thawed and drained

1 (15-ounce) can low-sodium
   tomatoes
¼ cup pitted and chopped black
   kalamata olives
1 teaspoon grated organic lemon
   zest
juice from one lemon
⅔ cup vegetable broth
2 teaspoons Bragg Liquid Amino
   Acids
4 small wild snapper fillets (4
   ounces each, cut in half if
   necessary)
20 ounces (4 bags) baby spinach
1 tablespoon cold-pressed olive oil

Preheat oven to 425 degrees.
Steam-sauté onion and garlic for
about 4 minutes. Add wine and
boil until completely reduced. Add
artichoke hearts, tomatoes, olives,
lemon zest, lemon juice, vegetable
broth, and Bragg, and simmer
uncovered over medium-high heat,
stirring occasionally, reducing
sauce, for 2 to 3 minutes. Rinse
fish and pat dry. Transfer sauce to a
3-quart baking dish. Arrange fish
(without crowding) over sauce.
Cover dish tightly with foil. Bake
fish about 12 to 14 minutes. While
fish is baking, steam spinach until
just wilted (about 2 minutes). Serve

fish on top of spinach beds.
Drizzle with olive oil and serve.

CITRUS SALMON WITH
GARLIC GREENS
Servings: 4

½ cup orange juice (fresh is better)
2 teaspoons organic orange zest
4 teaspoons Bragg Liquid Amino
   Acids
3 teaspoons (separated) minced or
   pressed garlic
4 (4-ounce) wild salmon fillets
   (about 1 inch thick), skinned
1 teaspoon cold-pressed virgin
   olive oil
20 ounces fresh organic baby
   spinach or four 5-ounce bags
1 tablespoon seasoned rice vinegar
½ teaspoon toasted sesame oil
¼ cup green onions, thinly sliced
   on the diagonal

Combine orange juice, zest,
Bragg, 2 teaspoons of garlic, and
salmon in sealable plastic bag.
Refrigerate for 30 minutes. Preheat
oven to 500 degrees. Remove
salmon from bag, and discard marinade. Lightly oil baking pan with
olive oil. Place salmon in baking
pan. Bake for 13 minutes or until
just cooked through. Steam
spinach with remaining teaspoon of

garlic until wilted, about 2 minutes. Remove from heat, and toss with vinegar and sesame oil. Arrange spinach on plate, and top with salmon and green onions.

WILD SALMON AND ASPARAGUS GREEN CURRY
Servings: 8

1½ pounds wild salmon fillet, skinned and cut in 2-inch pieces
2 whole red bell peppers, seeded and thinly sliced
3 pounds fresh asparagus, woody stems removed, cut in 2-inch diagonals
4 cups bok choy, cut in 1-inch crosswise slices
3 cups sliced shiitake and button mushrooms
1 can bamboo shoots, sliced
1 cup frozen peas
1 bunch fresh spinach (torn in pieces) or baby spinach
6 green onions, cut in 1-inch diagonals
4 cups cooked Wehani or brown rice

Sauce

4 cups carrot juice
½ cup unsweetened coconut milk
6 cloves garlic
2-inch piece fresh ginger root
6 sprigs fresh mint leaves
1 bunch basil
½ bunch cilantro leaves
2 teaspoons green curry paste
½ cup unsalted raw cashews
1 teaspoon Bragg Liquid Amino Acids

In blender, combine sauce ingredients (save some whole fresh herb sprigs for garnish and seasoning) and blend until very smooth. Place salmon chunks, vegetables (except for spinach and green onions), and sauce in wok or large skillet. Bring to a boil and simmer covered, stirring occasionally and gently, for about 5 to 10 minutes. Add spinach right before serving. Serve with a small portion of cooked rice, topped with green onions and herb sprigs.

Note: You can use a frozen Asian vegetable mix instead of fresh vegetables.

WILD SALMON SALAD NIÇOISE
Servings: 2

½ cup flaked salmon (wild, canned, or leftover)
2 cups green beans, cooked
1 cup red potatoes (with skins), cooked and cubed

½ cup chopped bell pepper, seeds removed

½ cup thinly sliced sweet onion

2 cups mixed salad greens (baby greens)

½ cucumber, cubed

1 tomato, coarsely chopped

2 cups romaine lettuce, torn in small pieces

Dressing

1 tablespoon fresh lemon juice

2 teaspoons Dijon mustard

1 tablespoon cold-pressed olive oil

2 teaspoons Bragg Liquid Amino Acids

2 tablespoons orange juice

1 teaspoon garlic powder

In a large salad bowl, combine salad ingredients. Whisk dressing ingredients, pour over salad, toss well, and serve.

SALMON VEGGIE WRAP
Servings: 2

⅔ cup flaked salmon (wild, canned, or leftover)

1 cup thinly shredded cabbage

1 tomato, chopped

½ cucumber, chopped

¼ cup thinly sliced onion

10 large leaf lettuce leaves

Dressing

1 cup tomato pasta sauce

2 tablespoons almond butter

1 tablespoon balsamic vinegar

1 tablespoon ketchup

1 teaspoon Bragg Liquid Amino Acids

Whisk dressing ingredients and add additional seasonings such as garlic or onion powder if you like. In a large salad bowl, toss salmon, cabbage, tomato, cucumber, and onion in generous portion of dressing. Spoon on lettuce leaves and roll up.

GRILLED RAINBOW TROUT WITH ROASTED VEGETABLES
Servings: 8

4 whole rainbow trout, boned and split in half (each trout makes 2 fillets)

1 clove garlic, pressed

juice of 1 lemon

1 tablespoon Worcestershire sauce

2 teaspoons Spike Salt-Free Seasoning

lemon or lime slices

½ cup chopped fresh parsley

Prepare Roasted Vegetables according to recipe in Side Dishes section, and keep warm in oven.

Marinate trout in garlic, lemon juice, Worcestershire, and a liberal sprinkling of Spike. Heat grill on high for at least 5 minutes with lid closed. Place trout skin-side down and close lid. Grill for 4 to 5 minutes until skin is crispy. Flip carefully and remove skin while on grill. Gently take off grill and place in a warmer or oven preheated to 175 degrees. Serve trout on top of bed of Roasted Vegetables with lemon or lime slices. Sprinkle with parsley.

GRILLED RAINBOW TROUT WITH SHALLOT-TOMATO SAUCE OVER FRESH GREENS
Servings: 8

4 whole rainbow trout, boned and split in half (each trout makes 2 fillets)
1 clove garlic, pressed
juice of 1 lemon
1 tablespoon Worcestershire sauce
2 teaspoons Spike Salt-Free Seasoning
8 Roma tomatoes, cut in ½-inch cubes
½ cup coarsely chopped shallots
2 teaspoons Bragg Liquid Amino Acids
1 teaspoon organic lemon zest
½ cup white table wine
¼ cup water

1 pound fresh baby salad mix
½ cup chopped parsley

Marinate trout in garlic, lemon juice, Worcestershire, and a liberal sprinkling of Spike. Heat grill on high for at least 5 minutes with lid closed. Place trout skin-side down and close lid. Grill for 4 to 5 minutes until skin is crispy. Flip carefully and remove skin while on grill. Gently remove from grill and place in a warmer or a warm oven.

Simmer tomatoes, shallots, Bragg, zest, white wine, and water until shallots are soft. Keep warm.

Portion salad greens equally on plate. Place fish on top of greens, spoon sauce over fish, sprinkle with fresh parsley, and serve.

VERY WILD SALMON SALAD
Servings: 6

Rice

¾ cup wild rice
½ cup brown rice
4 cups water

Salmon

½ cup dry white wine
1 cup water
½ lemon, sliced very thin
1 medium onion, sliced thin

3 tablespoons raisins

1 tablespoon pickling spices tied in
a cheesecloth bag

¾ pound wild salmon fillet, skin
removed by fishmonger

Salad

1 bunch watercress, coarse stems
discarded and sprigs chopped
coarse

½ cup coarsely chopped walnuts

2 teaspoons Bragg Liquid Amino
Acids

4 cups mixed baby greens, including
arugula

To prepare rice: Put rice and
water in a saucepan. Bring water to
a boil. Cover, turn heat to low, and
simmer for 45 minutes or until
done. Let rice rest, covered, for 10
minutes. Drain rice if water
remains.

To prepare salmon: In a medium
saucepan, combine liquids and
other listed ingredients except
salmon and 4 lemon slices, bring to
a boil, and simmer covered for 5
minutes to blend flavors. Place
salmon in cooking liquid. (Liquid
will not cover fish.) Poach salmon,
covered, for 7 minutes. Remove
salmon from liquid and chill.
Remove lemon, raisins, and onions

from cooking liquid and reserve all
ingredients except pickling spices.

Chop 4 reserved lemon slices.
In a large bowl, combine rice and
¼ cup cooking liquid. Break
salmon into large flakes and add to
bowl. Add chopped lemon, onions,
raisins, salmon, watercress, walnuts, and Bragg and toss mixture.
Serve on top of mixed greens.

WILD SALMON WITH ORANGE-GINGER RELISH OVER BRAISED BOK CHOY
Servings: 8

⅓ cup dry white wine

⅓ cup orange juice

4 teaspoons Bragg Liquid Amino
Acids

2 pounds wild salmon fillet, with
skin

6 cups bok choy, sliced crosswise
into 2-inch pieces

1 tablespoon unhulled sesame
seeds, lightly toasted

Relish

3 large navel oranges

1 cup thinly sliced red pepper

1 cup thinly sliced red onion

3 tablespoons chopped fresh
cilantro

3 teaspoons peeled and minced
fresh ginger

2 teaspoons grated orange peel
1 teaspoon Asian toasted sesame oil
¼ teaspoon dried crushed red pepper
2 teaspoons Bragg Liquid Amino
   Acids

Whisk first 3 ingredients in small bowl, then pour into 13x9x2-inch glass baking dish. Place salmon, skin-side down, in the liquid mixture. Cover with plastic and chill at least 2 hours and up to 4 hours.

To make relish: Use small sharp knife to peel oranges down to flesh. Working over bowl, cut between membranes to release segments into bowl. In medium bowl, combine the rest of the ingredients. Fold in reserved orange segments and any accumulated juices. (Can be prepared 1 hour ahead. Let stand at room temperature.)

Preheat oven to 450 degrees. Use nonstick baking pan and brush with vegetable oil. Place fish on prepared baking sheet. Bake until fish is just opaque and silky in center, about 15 to 20 minutes. Meanwhile, steam-sauté bok choy until tender, about 8 minutes. Keep warm.

Using large spatula, gently loosen salmon and remove skin (skin should come off easily). Place bed of bok choy on plate or platter. Place salmon on bok choy. Mound orange-ginger relish on center of fish, sprinkle with sesame seeds, and serve.

WILD SALMON PATTIES WITH FRESH TOMATO SALSA
Servings: 4

Salsa

2 large ripe tomatoes, peeled, seeded, and diced
3 green onions, chopped
1 clove garlic, peeled and minced
2 tablespoons chopped fresh parsley
2 teaspoons cold-pressed olive oil
1 teaspoon red wine vinegar
3 tablespoons chopped fresh basil
crushed red pepper

Salmon

1 pound fresh wild salmon fillet cut into ¼-inch pieces (ask fishmonger to remove skin)
2 egg whites, lightly beaten
½ cup whole-grain breadcrumbs
½ cup green onion, chopped
3 cloves garlic, pressed
2 teaspoons chopped fresh dill
3 tablespoons chopped fresh parsley

1 teaspoon Bragg Liquid Amino
   Acids
2 teaspoons cold-pressed olive oil
8 cups arugula, torn into bite-sized
   pieces
broccoli sprouts

Combine salsa ingredients in a
bowl, seasoning with crushed red
pepper to taste. Cover and set
aside.

For salmon patties, combine all
ingredients except oil and arugula
in a bowl. Mix well. Form ham-
burger-sized patties. In large nonstick frying pan, heat oil over
medium heat. Add patties and cook
4 minutes on each side until
cooked through.

Divide arugula among 4 plates.
Place one patty on each and top
with salsa and a pile of broccoli
sprouts.

BROILED ORANGE WILD SALMON
Servings: 6

1½ pounds wild salmon fillet, skin
   removed by fishmonger
½ cup fresh orange juice
¼ cup fresh lemon juice
1 teaspoon orange zest (from
   organic orange)

2 teaspoons Bragg Liquid Amino
   Acids
6 cloves garlic, pressed

Brush rimmed baking sheet
with a little oil and place salmon on
it. Mix orange juice, lemon juice,
zest, Bragg, and garlic in small
bowl; pour over salmon. Let stand
15 minutes. Preheat broiler. Broil
salmon, without turning fish over,
until just opaque and silky in center, about 12 minutes. Watch
closely and turn baking sheet once
for even broiling.

GRILLED SALMON AND
BEAN SALAD
Servings: 6

½ pound salmon (leftover grilled
   salmon is fine)
juice of 1 lemon (if grilling)
2 garlic cloves, pressed (if grilling)
olive oil spray (if grilling)
no-salt dried herb seasoning (if
   grilling)
3 red or yellow bell peppers, seeded
   and cut in ½-inch slices
juice of 2 large lemons, plus more
   to taste if necessary
3 cups cooked or canned white
   beans, drained
3 teaspoons cold-pressed olive oil

3 teaspoons Bragg Liquid Amino
Acids
10 cherry tomatoes, halved
1 medium sweet onion, thinly
sliced
6 kalamata olives, pitted and
coarsely chopped
¼ cup minced fresh basil leaves
¼ cup minced fresh parsley leaves
12 cups torn assorted salad greens

This is a great salad to make
when you have leftover grilled
salmon.

If you are starting with raw
salmon, start a charcoal or wood
fire or preheat a gas grill or broiler;
the rack should be about 4 inches
from the heat source. Marinate the
fish in lemon, garlic, herbal seasoning, and a small amount of olive oil
for 30 minutes. When the fire is
ready—it should be quite hot—
grill the fish for 3 to 4 minutes per
side.

If using leftover fish, skip the
preceding marinating and grilling
instructions. Grill the red pepper
slices. Cut the fish into small cubes
and toss it with the lemon juice,
beans, olive oil, and Bragg while
you prepare the other ingredients.
Add the tomatoes, onions, olives,
and herbs to the salmon. Taste for
seasoning and correct to your pref-

erence. Add lemon juice if necessary. Serve on a bed of greens,
topped with the strips of grilled red
pepper.

WILD SALMON PACKAGES WITH FENNEL, SWEET POTATOES, LEEKS, AND OLIVES
Servings: 6

2 small fennel bulbs, stalks
discarded
3 medium carrots
2 medium sweet potatoes
½ cup kalamata olives, slivered
2 teaspoons organic lemon zest
4 teaspoons fresh thyme
4 large garlic cloves, minced or
pressed
3 teaspoons Bragg Liquid Amino
Acids
2 teaspoons Worcestershire sauce
2 teaspoons cold-pressed olive oil
1½ pounds wild salmon fillet,
skinned and cut into 6 pieces
no-salt seasoning (your choice)
6 (15-inch) squares parchment
paper
kitchen string

Place a large baking sheet on
bottom rack of oven and remove
any other racks. Preheat oven to
400 degrees. Halve fennel bulbs
lengthwise. Remove most of core,

leaving enough intact to keep layers together when sliced. Cut fennel bulbs (lengthwise), carrots (diagonally), and sweet potatoes into ⅛-inch-thick slices. Steam-sauté vegetables, adding water as needed to keep from scorching, until almost tender, 8 to 10 minutes. Remove from heat; add olives, zest, thyme, half of garlic, Bragg, Worcestershire, and olive oil; and toss together.

Place salmon in center of parchment square. Evenly distribute vegetable mixture on top of salmon. Season with any no-salt seasoning of your choice. Gather sides of parchment up over vegetable mixture to form a pouch, leaving no openings, and tie tightly with string. Place packages directly on hot baking sheet in oven and cook 20 minutes. Serve immediately.

SAUTÉED WILD SALMON
Servings: 4

1 pound wild salmon fillet, skin removed by fishmonger
1 lime
1 clove garlic, pressed
2 teaspoons Spike Salt-Free Seasoning

Squeeze lime on salmon, spread salmon with garlic, and sprinkle with Spike. Heat heavy large skillet over medium-high heat. Add salmon and sauté until just opaque and silky in the center, about 5 minutes per side. Transfer fish to plates.

Note: Delicious served on top of lightly dressed tossed salad.

Free-Range Poultry

AFRICAN GROUND-NUT CHICKEN-OKRA STEW
Servings: 10

2 tablespoons tomato paste
½ cup smooth unsalted peanut butter, room temperature
4 teaspoons Bragg Liquid Amino Acids
4 cups carrot juice
4 boned and skinned chicken breast halves, cut into bite-sized pieces
2 cups chopped frozen onion
1 (15-oz) can whole no-salt crushed tomatoes (San Marzano are the sweetest)
4 garlic cloves, minced or pressed
3 teaspoons chili powder (4 if you like it spicier)
1 pinch cayenne pepper
1 medium sweet potato

16 ounces frozen okra, thawed and cut in half crosswise

16 ounces chopped frozen kale or collard greens

1½ cups fresh or frozen (thawed) fruit (apples, berries, pears, peaches, or your choice)

Whisk tomato paste, peanut butter, Bragg, and carrot juice in large saucepan. Add the rest of the ingredients. Mix together, bring to a boil, cover and simmer on low heat for about 40 minutes. Serve topped with fruit.

INDIAN VEGETABLE CHICKEN CURRY
Servings: 8

2 free-range chicken breasts, boned and skinned

1 onion, chopped

1 green bell pepper, seeded and chopped

8 garlic cloves, pressed or minced

2 tablespoons curry powder

2 teaspoons garam masala (dried, ground spice mix found in Indian or health food stores)

1½ teaspoons chili powder

2 cups canned chopped Italian plum tomatoes

2 cups water

2 teaspoons Bragg Liquid Amino Acids

4 carrots, halved lengthwise and cut in ½-inch pieces

2 sweet potatoes, peeled and cubed

1 cauliflower, trimmed and cut into small florets

1 cinnamon stick

2 (15-ounce) cans garbanzo beans, rinsed and drained

3 tablespoons currants

4 cups cooked quinoa or brown rice

½ cup raw cashew pieces

¼ cup chopped cilantro

Using a sharp knife, slice raw chicken breast crosswise in thin slices. Spray skillet with olive oil. Sauté the chicken over medium-high heat for about 5 minutes, or until the chicken is sealed on all sides and starting to brown. Set aside.

In large pot, combine all ingredients except for chicken, garbanzo beans, currants, rice, cashews, and cilantro. Cover and simmer for about 20 minutes, until all vegetables are tender. Stir in chicken, garbanzo beans, and currants, and cook for five minutes longer. Remove cinnamon stick, and serve with quinoa or brown rice. Sprinkle with cilantro and cashew pieces.

GARLIC CHICKEN AND COLLARDS STIR-FRY
Servings: 4

1 teaspoon cold-pressed olive oil
2 boneless chicken breasts, sliced in very thin strips
4 garlic cloves, pressed
1 green bell pepper, seeded and cut in thin strips
1 red bell pepper, seeded and cut in thin strips
1 onion, sliced
1½ cups Chinese pea pods or sugar snap peas
4 cups shredded collard greens
1 (15-ounce) can adzuki or red beans, rinsed and drained
¼ cup raw cashew nuts
4 green onions, chopped for garnish

Sauce

2 cups carrot juice
3 tablespoons peanut butter
1-inch slice fresh ginger
6 cloves garlic, cut in half
2 teaspoons Bragg Liquid Amino Acids

Blend the sauce ingredients in a blender and set aside.

Oil wok with olive oil and heat. Add chicken and stir-fry for about 3 to 4 minutes until chicken is cooked through. Add garlic, vegetables, and beans and steam-sauté with water as needed to keep from scorching for 5 minutes. Stir in the sauce and heat through until mixture starts to bubble. Serve topped with cashews and chopped green onion.

ROTISSERIE CHICKEN-APPLE SALAD
Servings: 4

1 rotisserie chicken, breast meat only
6 sun-dried tomatoes, reconstituted
1 tablespoon cold-pressed virgin olive oil
½ bunch parsley plus 1 teaspoon chopped
1 tablespoon tahini
1 tablespoon fresh lemon juice
2 tablespoons water
2 teaspoons Bragg Liquid Amino Acids
2 Granny Smith apples, peeled and cut into julienne strips
½ cup chopped walnuts
1 teaspoon chopped fresh basil
8 large Boston lettuce leaves

Shred chicken breasts. Puree sun-dried tomatoes with oil, ½ bunch parsley, tahini, lemon juice, water, and Bragg. Toss apples and pureed sauce together with walnuts and basil. Place 2 lettuce leaves per plate. Mound with apple salad, and top with shredded chicken. Sprinkle with remaining parsley.

BAKED BLUEBERRY-GARLIC CHICKEN
Servings: 6

4 Granny Smith apples, peeled and quartered
½ fresh pineapple, peeled and quartered
2 organic oranges, quartered and seeded
1 onion, peeled and quartered
½ bunch fresh thyme
8 fresh sage leaves
6 small chicken breasts, skinned with bones
½ cup blueberry 100% fruit spread
2 teaspoons Bragg Liquid Amino Acids
6 cloves garlic, pressed
3 teaspoons Spike Salt-Free Seasoning or other no-salt herb seasoning
chopped parsley for garnish

Preheat oven to 350 degrees. In baking pan arrange apples, pineapple, oranges, and onion close together. Spread sage and thyme over fruit mixture. Place breasts, bone-side down, on top of that. In a small bowl, combine blueberry spread, Bragg, garlic, and Spike. Generously spread this mixture over chicken. Cover with foil and bake for about 30 to 40 minutes, depending on weight of chicken or until juices run clear when pricked to center with a fork. Garnish with parsley.

VEGETABLE STRATA WITH TOMATO SALSA
Servings: 12

olive oil
1 large leek or onion, sliced thin
5 cloves garlic, pressed or minced
1 pound frozen broccoli florets
1 large red bell pepper, seeded and sliced thin (about 2 cups)
1 teaspoon dried Herbes de Provence (French dried herbs)
6 ounces fresh spinach or 1 bag baby spinach
12 slices multigrain bread, cut into ¾-inch squares
4 ounces mozzarella cheese substitute (Soya Kaas), shredded
2 large eggs (free-range)
whites from 10 large eggs (free-range)
2½ cups unsweetened soy milk
½ cup chopped fresh parsley or 2 tablespoons dried
¼ teaspoon red pepper flakes
2 cups tomato salsa

Lightly oil a 2½-quart baking dish, 13x9x2 inches, with cooking spray. In a large nonstick skillet, water-sauté onion and 1 tablespoon garlic, broccoli, bell peppers, and Herbes de Provence. Cook covered over low heat for 5 minutes. Add water as necessary to prevent scorching. Add spinach and cook until wilted. Spread bread squares evenly in baking dish and top with vegetables. Sprinkle ½ cup soy mozzarella evenly over vegetables. In a bowl, whisk together whole eggs, egg whites, soy milk, parsley, any vegetable liquid, and pepper flakes. Pour evenly over bread and vegetables. Chill strata, covered, for at least 3 hours and up to 12. Preheat oven to 350 degrees and let strata stand at room temperature for 20 minutes. Bake in middle of oven for 45 to 55 minutes, or until puffed and golden brown around edges. Serve strata topped with fresh tomato salsa.

CURRIED CHICKEN WITH FRUITS
Servings: 4

2 chicken breasts, skinless and
  boneless
2 onions, chopped

2 teaspoons garlic powder or 2
  minced or pressed fresh garlic
  cloves
3 teaspoons curry powder
¼ teaspoon cumin
1 teaspoon turmeric
½ teaspoon coriander powder
1½ cups carrot juice
2 cans diced tomatoes, no salt
2 Granny Smith apples, peeled,
  cored, and quartered
½ cup currants
½ cup goji berries (optional)
2 teaspoons Bragg Liquid Amino
  Acids
pinch of crushed red pepper, or to
  taste
2 teaspoons grated ginger root
10 ounces baby spinach
1 cup cooked brown rice
¼ cup chopped fresh cilantro and
  green onions

Slice raw chicken breast very thin. In wok or large skillet, simmer onions, garlic, curry powder, cumin, turmeric, and coriander in carrot juice until tender, about 15 minutes. Add chicken and simmer until chicken begins to firm up and lighten, about 3 minutes. Add tomatoes, apples, currants, goji berries, Bragg, red pepper, and ginger. Bring to a boil then reduce heat and simmer, covered, for about 10 minutes. Serve over a bed of baby spinach and ¼ cup cooked rice. Top with chopped fresh cilantro and green onions.

QUICK CARROT CHICKEN STIR-FRY
Servings: 4

2 skinless and boneless chicken
   breasts, thinly sliced
4 cloves garlic, cut in half
½ bunch chopped cilantro
   (optional)
12 fresh basil leaves
½ bunch chopped fresh mint
1 slice (½ inch) fresh ginger
2½ cups carrot juice
2½ teaspoons arrowroot powder
3 teaspoons Bragg Liquid Amino
   Acids
½ teaspoon curry powder
   (optional)
3 tablespoons unsalted peanut or
   raw cashew butter
½ cup light coconut milk
2 (16-ounce) bags frozen Asian
   vegetables
1 onion, sliced
½ pound sliced mushrooms
1 (16-ounce) bag broccoli florets
1 can bamboo shoots, drained
2 cups cooked brown rice or
   quinoa
¼ cup chopped raw cashews

In blender, finely chop garlic, cilantro, basil, mint, and ginger, then blend in arrowroot, Bragg, curry, nut butter, and coconut milk. Place all ingredients except the rice and cashews into a wok or large skillet. Cook on high heat, covered, stirring often, until vegetables are just tender and chicken is cooked through, about 10 to 15 minutes. Serve with rice or quinoa (high-protein grain found in health food stores), topped with chopped cashews. Also delicious topped with the fresh herbs.

CARROT-CITRUS CHICKEN
Servings: 4

2 bunches kale
2 skinless and boneless chicken
   breasts, halved
Spike Salt-Free Seasoning
2 cups fresh carrot juice
1½ teaspoons organic lemon zest
4 cloves garlic, minced or pressed
1 tablespoon minced ginger root
2 teaspoons Bragg Liquid Amino
   Acids (optional)
1 cup orange juice
1½ tablespoons arrowroot or
   cornstarch
½ cup chopped parsley

Steam kale for 20 minutes. Coat chicken breast with Spike. Lightly oil pan with olive oil and heat pan. Lightly brown chicken over high heat. Turn and brown on other side. Turn down heat to medium and cook until slightly underdone. Do not overcook chicken; when pricked with fork, the juice should run slightly pink, almost clear. Remove to a plate and set aside.

Using the same pan, combine carrot juice, lemon zest, garlic, and Bragg and simmer on high heat for 5 minutes to reduce sauce. Mix arrowroot with orange juice and add to simmering sauce. Add chicken to sauce and cover for 3 minutes. Serve chicken and sauce atop a bed of steamed kale. Garnish with fresh parsley.

CHICKEN BREASTS WITH LEEK-AND-WILD-MUSHROOM STUFFING
Servings: 6

3 chicken breasts, skinned and with bone in
1 teaspoon Bragg Liquid Amino Acids
2 teaspoons no-salt herb seasoning
½ cup hot water
1 ounce dried porcini mushrooms (other dried mushrooms are fine)
1 pound fresh shiitake mushrooms, stems removed and caps sliced
1 pound button mushrooms, sliced
1 cup no-salt chicken broth
1½ cups chopped leeks (white and pale green parts only)
6 garlic cloves, chopped
2 cups dry white wine
1 tablespoon chopped fresh thyme
6 slices whole-grain bread (Ezekiel or Genesis is great), torn in small pieces
½ cup chopped walnuts
2 tablespoons 100% fruit or berry spread
1 cup chopped parsley

Rinse chicken breast, brush with Bragg, season with half of the no-salt herb seasoning, and return to refrigerator. Combine hot water and dried porcini in small bowl. Let stand until mushrooms soften, about 30 minutes, or microwave for 1 minute. Preheat oven to 350 degrees. Using slotted spoon, transfer mushrooms to work surface; chop finely. In heavy large pot over medium-high heat, combine porcini mushrooms, shiitake and button mushrooms, and broth; steam-sauté for 5 minutes. Add leeks and garlic; sauté an additional 5 minutes. Add wine and thyme. Cook until almost all wine evaporates, stirring occasionally, about 5 minutes. Transfer mixture to very large bowl. Mix bread and nuts into mushroom mixture. Season with rest of no-salt herb seasoning. Lightly spray a glass baking dish with olive oil. Transfer stuffing to prepared dish. Place chicken breasts on top of stuffing and spread with fruit or berry spread. Lightly cover with foil. Bake 30 to 45 minutes or until chicken juices run clear when pricked with a fork. Served garnished with parsley.

Note: Dried porcini mushrooms are available at Italian markets, specialty food stores, and many supermarkets.

VEGETABLE CHICKEN SOUP WITH BASIL-GARLIC PISTOU
Servings: 8

Soup
1 small fennel bulb (sometimes called anise)
2 chicken breasts, skinned with bone in
1 medium onion, chopped
4 cups kale, de-stemmed and torn in pieces
3 medium carrots, peeled and cut in ½-inch pieces
¼ small cabbage, cored and chopped (2 cups)

6 cups water
4 cups no- or low-sodium chicken broth
1 (10-ounce) package frozen baby lima beans
½ lb fresh or frozen green beans, trimmed and cut in 1-inch pieces
2 small zucchinis, cut into ½-inch pieces
1 medium sweet potato, peeled and cut into ½-inch pieces
2 sprigs fresh thyme
1 bay leaf
1 (15-ounce) can cannellini or other white beans, drained and rinsed
5 ounces baby spinach (5 cups)

Pistou
3 large garlic cloves
1½ cups fresh basil leaves
½ cup walnuts
1 tablespoon cold-pressed olive oil
3 tablespoons Romano cheese

For soup, cut fennel stalks flush with bulb, discarding stalks, and trim off any tough outer layers from bulb. Chop fennel into ½-inch pieces. In soup kettle, combine chicken, fennel, onion, kale, carrots, cabbage, water, and broth and simmer, uncovered, 30 minutes. Add lima beans, green beans, summer squash, sweet potato, thyme, bay leaf, and cannellini beans; simmer until vegetables are tender, about 5 to 10 minutes. Discard thyme sprigs and bay leaf. Remove chicken and cool for a few minutes. Shred chicken by hand and return to soup.

Prepare pistou while soup is simmering. Blend pistou ingredients in blender or food processor until finely chopped, a coarse paste. Stir spinach into hot soup to wilt. Serve topped with a teaspoon of pistou.

Grass-Fed Red Meat

BISON FILLETS WITH MUSHROOM-PEPPER WINE SAUCE
Servings: 2

10 ounces grass-fed lean bison tenderloin steaks—2 fillets cut in half for 4 servings
4 cloves garlic, pressed
juice of 1 lemon or lime
2 teaspoons Worcestershire sauce
½ teaspoon low-sodium soy sauce

Sauce
1 medium red bell pepper, seeded and sliced in strips
¼ pound shiitake mushrooms, sliced

2 large portobello mushrooms, sliced
¼ pound button mushrooms, sliced
2 cloves garlic, pressed
½ cup chopped fresh parsley
2 teaspoons Bragg Liquid Amino Acids
1 teaspoon dried Herbes de Provence or Italian seasoning mix
½ cup water
¼ cup red wine

Mix 4 garlic cloves, lime juice, Worcestershire, and soy. Pour over steaks, marinate for 1 hour. Broil to your desired doneness. Simmer all sauce ingredients until liquid is reduced and mushrooms are tender and juicy. Serve steaks with mushroom wine sauce.

Wild Game

SMOKEY VENISON VEGETABLE GOULASH
Servings: 10

2 pounds venison stew meat (or free-range chicken breast or free-range buffalo stew meat)
6 onions, chopped
1 carrot, chopped

2 red bell peppers, seeded and
chopped
8 garlic cloves, pressed
1 teaspoon caraway seed
2 cups prepared tomato soup, no
salt (Health Valley makes one)
1 (24-ounce) can crushed tomatoes, no added salt
6 cups water
1 cube Rapunzel Salt-Free Bouillon
(optional)
1 tablespoon Bragg Liquid Amino
Acids
6 cups shredded cabbage
2 pounds mushrooms (preferably
white and shiitake), sliced
3 tablespoons sweet Hungarian
paprika
2 teaspoons smoked paprika (add
more for additional smoky flavor)
fat-free plain yogurt
chopped fresh parsley for garnish

Spray bottom of soup kettle
with oil and lightly brown venison.
Add onions, carrot, bell peppers,
garlic, caraway seed, tomato soup,
crushed tomatoes, water, bouillon,
and Bragg. Cover and simmer over
low heat for 2 to 3 hours or until
venison is tender. Add remaining
ingredients and simmer covered for
30 minutes. Serve with a dollop of
fat-free plain yogurt and parsley as
garnish.

POMEGRANATE BAKED WILD QUAIL OR DOVES WITH FIGS, CURRANTS, AND RED CABBAGE
Servings: 4

1 pomegranate
4 cups shredded red cabbage
2 onions, thinly sliced
6 cloves garlic, pressed
1 cup dried figs, halved with stems
removed
½ cup dried currants
1 tablespoon Worcestershire sauce
½ cup bottled pomegranate juice
½ cup red wine
1 cup chicken broth
4 teaspoons Bragg Liquid Amino
Acids
1 tablespoon chopped fresh
tarragon
½ teaspoon dried thyme
1 organic orange with peel, cut into
quarters
8 dressed quail or doves
1 tablespoon cold-pressed olive oil
½ cup chopped parsleys for garnish
½ cup pine nuts

Pull pomegranate apart.
Remove seeds in a bowl of water;
seeds will sink to the bottom, skin
and white flesh will float. Reserve
seeds for later. Preheat oven to 350
degrees for regular baking dish. For
Romertopf, do not preheat oven,
place clay vessel in cold oven, and

bake dish at 400 degrees. In soaked clay pot or covered baking dish, combine and mix all ingredients except for birds, olive oil, pomegranate seeds, parsley, and pine nuts. In skillet, brown birds in olive oil. Place birds on top of cabbage mixture. For baking dish: Cover and bake for 1 hour. For clay pot: Cover and bake for 1 hour 15 minutes. Remove orange and serve sprinkled with fresh pomegranate seeds, parsley, and pine nuts.

AUSTRIAN WILD PHEASANT WITH RED CABBAGE
Servings: 6

Pheasant

2-pound pheasant
¼ teaspoon allspice
6 cloves garlic, pressed
1 cup dry red wine
3 teaspoons Bragg Liquid Amino Acids
½ tablespoon olive oil

Rice

½ cup wild rice, uncooked
1 cup salt-free chicken broth
1 (3-inch) sprig fresh rosemary

Cabbage

1 onion, sliced thin
6 cups red cabbage(about ½ head), thinly sliced
2 teaspoons balsamic vinegar
¾ cup orange juice
1 bay leaf
½ teaspoon sea salt
¼ teaspoon cracked red pepper
¼ teaspoon ground allspice
⅓ cup currants
¼ cup (about 3) minced shallots
⅔ cup dry white wine
½ cup halved red and/or green seedless grapes
3 Granny Smith apples, peeled and coarsely chopped

Rinse pheasant under cold water and pat dry inside and out. Cut pheasant into 6 serving pieces. In plastic bag, marinate pheasant in allspice, garlic, red wine, and Bragg for at least 30 minutes.

Preheat oven to 350 degrees.

In a strainer, rinse wild rice well and drain. In a covered flameproof casserole, place rice, broth, and rosemary. Bake covered for 1 hour, or until liquid is absorbed and rice is tender. This can be cooked at the same time as the pheasant.

In a separate casserole, combine all the cabbage ingredients. Remove pheasant from marinade and pat dry. In a heavy skillet, heat oil and sauté pheasant until golden, about 5 minutes on each side. Place browned pheasant on top of cabbage mixture, cover, and bake for 2½ to 3 hours until breast meat is tender. Serve pheasant and cabbage with the wild rice.

CLAY POT COOKING

Baking foods in terracotta pots is an ancient tradition, dating back to Roman times. The pots were first soaked in water to create a moist cooking environment, thus eliminating the need for excess oils. The tightly closed, moist clay pot keeps the food very moist, seals in nutrients, and causes a delightful mingling of flavors. This is a delicious and healthy super antioxidant cooking technique.

Make sure you follow the manufacturer's instructions to prevent damage to your clay pot. The first step before preparing food in your clay pot is soaking. In your sink, completely submerge in water both the pot and lid and soak for 15 to 30 minutes.

Note: Always put your clay pot into a cold oven, then set the temperature.

CLAY POT VEGETABLE RAGOUT
Serves: 4

4 leeks, sliced in ¼-inch rounds
2 celery stalks, sliced
2 sweet potatoes, cut in ½-inch cubes
2 carrots, sliced in rounds
2 parsnips, sliced in rounds
½ cauliflower broken into florets
1½ cups cooked or canned garbanzo beans
3 cups shiitake mushrooms, sliced
2 tablespoons tomato paste
1 cup vegetable broth
1 tablespoon date sugar
2 teaspoons Bragg Liquid Amino Acids
1 bay leaf
4 tablespoons whole-grain breadcrumbs
4 tablespoons unhulled sesame seeds

Combine all ingredients, except breadcrumbs and sesame seeds, and turn into soaked pot. Cover the pot and place in cold oven. Set the oven at 425 degrees. Bake for 1 hour. Remove lid and stir ingredients. Sprinkle seeds and breadcrumbs over the top and bake uncovered for an additional 15 minutes, or until topping is golden and vegetables tender.

CLAY POT RATATOUILLE
Servings: 6

2 eggplants, cubed
2 teaspoons Bragg Liquid Amino
    Acids
1 green bell pepper, seeded and cut
    in ½-inch pieces
1 red bell pepper, seeded and cut in
    ½-inch pieces
1 pound mushrooms, sliced
1 large onion, halved and sliced
4 garlic cloves, crushed
1 teaspoon dried marjoram
½ pound zucchini, cut in 1-inch cubes
2 pounds tomatoes, peeled and
    quartered
1 bay leaf
½ cup chopped parsley

Combine all ingredients, except parsley, and turn into soaked clay pot. Cover the pot and place in cold oven. Set the oven temperature at 425 degrees. Cook for 1 hour and remove from oven. Leave uncovered outside of oven for 20 minutes before serving. Mix in parsley and serve.

CLAY POT MINESTRONE
Servings: 6

½ pound dried cannellini or Great
    Northern beans, soaked overnight
½ pound fresh or dried fava
    beans—if dry, soak overnight
1 large onion, chopped
6 cloves garlic, crushed
2 carrots, diced
2 medium sweet potatoes, diced
4 cups low-sodium canned diced
    tomatoes
4 cups shredded cabbage
3 cups shredded kale
2 bay leaves
2 teaspoons dried marjoram
1 tablespoon tomato paste
2 teaspoons Bragg Liquid Amino
    Acids
½ cube Rapunzel Salt-Free
    Vegetable Bouillon (optional)
¼ cup whole-grain spiral pasta
½ cup chopped parsley
½ cup chopped fresh basil
¼ cup pine nuts

Drain cannellini beans (and dried fava beans), place in a saucepan, and cover with water. Boil rapidly for 20 minutes. Drain beans and place in soaked clay pot. Combine all ingredients except pasta, parsley, basil, and pine nuts. Pour in 2½ quarts water. Cover pot and place in cold oven. Set oven at 400 degrees. Bake for 1½ hours or until beans are tender. Add pasta and bake for another 30 minutes, or until pasta is tender. Stir in fresh parsley and basil and serve topped with pine nuts.

CLAY POT DILLED SALMON ON VEGETABLES
Servings: 6

2 pounds sweet potatoes or yams, peeled and cut into 1-inch cubes
3 carrots, thinly sliced
3 small zucchini, thinly sliced
3 small yellow summer squash, thinly sliced
2 leeks, thinly sliced
grated rind and juice of 1 organic lime
1¼ pounds wild salmon, skinned and cut into 6 portions
6 cloves garlic, pressed
2 teaspoons Bragg Liquid Amino Acids
1 tablespoon chopped dill
2 teaspoons salt-free Spike or other dry herb seasoning
1½ cups frozen shelled peas, thawed

In saucepan, cook sweet potatoes and carrots for 8 to 10 minutes, until almost tender. Drain and place in the soaked clay pot. Add the zucchini, squash, leeks, and lime rind to vegetables in the clay pot. Mix well.

Arrange the salmon on top of the vegetables in the clay pot. Spread the salmon with pressed garlic, and Bragg and sprinkle with dill, lime juice, and Spike or dry herb seasoning. Cover the clay pot and place in cold oven. Set oven at 425 degrees. Bake for 30 minutes. Add the peas, sprinkling them on top of fish and vegetables. Bake for another 5 to 10 minutes until salmon is cooked and vegetables are tender.

CLAY POT WINTER SQUASH WITH VENISON SAUSAGE
Servings: 4

1 large onion, finely chopped
1½ pounds winter squash or pumpkin flesh, cubed
¼ pound venison sausage
2 teaspoons Bragg Liquid Amino Acids
½ pound shiitake mushrooms, sliced
½ pound small mushrooms
2 bay leaves
4 sprigs fresh thyme
2 avocados, cubed
juice of 1 lime
1 teaspoon date sugar
4 tablespoons pumpkin seeds, lightly roasted

Combine all ingredients except avocado, lime, date sugar, and pumpkin seeds in soaked clay pot. Cover the pot and place in cold oven. Set the oven at 425 degrees. Bake for 1 hour, or until squash is tender. Combine and mash avocado, lime juice, and date sugar. Serve squash dish topped with avocado mixture and pumpkin seeds.

CLAY POT BRANDIED FRUIT CHICKEN
Servings: 4–6

4 chicken breasts, boned and skinned
½ teaspoon ground mace
2 teaspoons Spike Salt-Free Seasoning
¼ pound pearl onions (frozen are fine)
4 tablespoons brandy
1 cup dry white wine
2 teaspoons Bragg Liquid Amino Acids
4 cloves garlic, chopped
½ pound unsulphured dried apricots
¼ pound unsulphured dried prunes, pitted
4 bay leaves
½ pound shiitake mushrooms, sliced

6 cups kale, destemmed and torn into bite-sized pieces
1 onion, coarsely chopped
4 cloves garlic, pressed

Sprinkle chicken breasts with mace and Spike. Brown in slightly oiled skillet. Place browned chicken in soaked clay pot. Brown the onions in chicken skillet. Pour in brandy, wine, and Bragg and then bring to a boil stirring. Add the chopped garlic, apricots, prunes, bay leaf, and mushrooms. Stir well and pour over chicken. Cover the pot and place in cold oven. Set oven to 425 degrees and cook for 1 hour. Steam-sauté kale, onion, and pressed garlic for 15 minutes until tender. Serve chicken over steamed kale.

CLAY POT WINTER FRUIT DELIGHT
Servings: 8

6 Granny Smith apples, peeled and sliced
8 dates, pitted and chopped
1 cup currants or raisins
1 cup frozen cherries
1 cup frozen blueberries
¼ cup water
¾ cup chopped walnuts or pecans
½ teaspoon cinnamon

¼ teaspoon nutmeg
2 cardamom pods
juice of 1 orange
2 teaspoons organic lemon zest
2 tablespoons brandy (optional)

Combine all ingredients in soaked clay pot, cover, and place in a cold oven. Set oven to 375 degrees and bake for 1 hour or until fruit is tender. Remove cardamom pods, stir in brandy, and serve.

Note: This dish is also good served cold.

SIDE DISHES

GARLIC-LEMON SPINACH
Servings: 4

2 cloves garlic, pressed
1¼ pounds fresh spinach or 4 bags baby spinach, stemmed
1 teaspoon cold-pressed olive oil
2 teaspoons organic lemon zest
4 tablespoons pine nuts

Steam spinach and garlic until spinach is just wilted, about 3 minutes. Place in bowl and toss with remaining ingredients.

TRACEY'S CASHEW-PEANUT STEW
Servings: 4–6

1 medium onion, chopped
6 cloves garlic, pressed
olive oil spray
2 tablespoons unsalted peanut butter
2 tablespoons raw cashew butter
1 tablespoon Tabasco
4 teaspoons Bragg Liquid Amino Acids
2 teaspoons Spike Salt-Free Seasoning
2 bunches kale (or 1 bunch kale and 1 bunch Swiss chard)
1 fresh pineapple, peeled and chopped
1 cup Sambazon Super Greens drink (or pineapple juice)
1 bunch fresh cilantro, chopped
½ cup chopped scallions
¼ cup chopped cashews

In large skillet or wok, steam-sauté onions and garlic until tender. Add nut butters, Tabasco, Bragg, and Spike and stir until mixed. In crock pot, combine all ingredients. Cook on low for 1 to 1½ hours until kale is tender. Top with scallions and cashews.

ASIAN MIXED VEGETABLES
Servings: 4

6 large garlic cloves, coarsely
   chopped
1 tablespoon white miso
1 pound assorted vegetables (such
   as broccoli, green beans, bok
   choy, eggplant, mushrooms, bell
   pepper—seeded, and bean
   sprouts), cut into bite-sized
   pieces; or use frozen mixed
   Asian or Oriental vegetables
1 jalapeño chili, seeded and thinly
   sliced
1½ cups water
¼ cup raw cashews
1 teaspoon toasted sesame oil

In wok or large frying pan,
combine all ingredients except
cashews and sesame oil. Steam-
sauté in water, covering and stirring, until vegetables are
crisp-tender and water has evaporated, about 12 minutes. Toss with
cashews and sesame oil, and serve.

BROCCOLI IN ORANGE SAUCE
Servings: 4

2 pounds broccoli florets
⅔ cup orange juice
2 tablespoons date sugar
1 teaspoon Dijon mustard

1 teaspoon organic orange zest
2 teaspoons white miso
1 clove garlic, crushed
⅛ teaspoon red pepper flakes
1½ teaspoons cornstarch or 3 teaspoons arrowroot powder
1 tablespoon water
1 teaspoon toasted sesame seeds

Trim the broccoli florets into
pieces about 1½ inches. Steam-
sauté for 5 minutes or until tender.
In a small saucepan over medium-
high heat, bring the orange juice,
date sugar, mustard, zest, miso,
garlic, and pepper flakes to a boil.
In small bowl, whisk together the
cornstarch and water. Stir into the
orange juice mixture and cook until
thickened, about 1 minute. Gently
toss the broccoli with the sauce to
coat. Sprinkle with sesame seeds.

AROMATIC SPICE AND HERB
BUTTERNUT SQUASH
Servings: 4

1 medium (or 2 small) butternut
   squash
powdered cinnamon
1 bulb garlic, slice ¼ inch off top
   of bulb
2 teaspoons fresh or dried herbs,
   any kind (thyme, marjoram,
   oregano, basil, mint)

at oven to 350 degrees. sh in half lengthwise. Scrape out and discard seeds. Sprinkle cavity generously with cinnamon and place garlic pod and herbs inside. Put squash back together and place in baking pan. Bake for 45 minutes to 1 hour depending on size, until tender.

ROASTED VEGETABLES
Servings: 6

½ pound fresh or frozen Brussels
   sprouts
½ pound baby carrots, cut in ½-
   inch slices
1 pound small broccoli florets
   (frozen is fine)
1 pound small cauliflower florets
   (frozen is fine)
1 red bell pepper, seeded and cut in
   bite-sized pieces
3 teaspoons cold-pressed olive oil
2 tablespoons balsamic vinegar
2 teaspoons Bragg Liquid Amino
   Acids, or use low-sodium soy sauce
6 cloves garlic, minced

Preheat oven to 450 degrees. If using fresh Brussels sprouts, cut off stem base, peel outer leaves, and cut a cross ¼-inch deep on base of stem. In a large bowl, combine all ingredients and toss.

Spread evenly on a large baking pan. Bake for 45 minutes, stirring every 15 minutes, or until the vegetables are slightly browned and tender. If they begin to get too brown before they are tender, pile them up to keep them moist, turn heat down to 350, and finish cooking.

Note: You can marinate vegetables before baking. I sometimes prep them the day before and marinate for 24 hours.

TUSCAN KALE-MUSHROOM SAUTÉ
Servings: 4

½ ounce dried porcini mushrooms
1 pound fresh mushrooms (any
   kind)
4 cups kale, de-stemmed and
   coarsely chopped
4 cloves of garlic, minced
½ onion, chopped
2 cups carrot juice or water
1 teaspoon Bragg Liquid Amino
   Acids
1 red bell pepper, seeded and cut
   into bite-sized pieces
1 can pinto beans, rinsed
2 cups coarsely chopped tomatoes
2 tablespoons pine nuts

Place dried mushrooms in a bowl with enough hot water to barely cover and let them soak for about 20 minutes. Wipe clean and slice the fresh mushrooms and remove any tough stems; set aside. In a large pan with a cover, simmer the kale, garlic, onion, Bragg, carrot juice, and dried mushrooms with soaking liquid for 15 minutes or until kale is almost tender. Add fresh mushrooms, red bell pepper, and beans, simmering on medium-high for 10 more minutes, stirring occasionally. Add water if necessary to keep from scorching. Add fresh tomatoes and gently toss until hot through. Serve sprinkled with pine nuts.

Note: Use as many different fresh mushrooms as you can find, especially the healthier varieties like shiitake, enoki, and oyster mushrooms. The dried porcini add a robust flavor. You'll find them in little packages near the produce stands in supermarkets. Asian markets often have a great assortment of exotic mushrooms at a reasonable price.

STEAMED BROCCOLI-GARLIC-RED BELL PEPPER MEDLEY
Servings: 3

1 head broccoli, small florets, with peeled and sliced ½-inch thick stems

1 red bell pepper, seeded and thinly sliced
6 garlic cloves, pressed or minced
½ cup water
1 can cannellini or navy beans, rinsed and drained
1 teaspoon cold-pressed olive oil
½ cup pine nuts, lightly toasted

In large saucepan, combine all ingredients except olive oil and pine nuts. Steam about 10 minutes or until broccoli is just tender. Add more water if necessary to keep from scorching. Toss with olive oil and top with pine nuts.

CASHEW MASHED CAULIFLOWER WITH LEEKS AND MUSHROOMS
Servings: 6

2 heads cauliflower, florets
10 cloves garlic, sliced
2 leeks, coarsely chopped
1 red bell pepper, seeded and coarsely chopped
½ pound shiitake mushrooms, sliced
⅛ teaspoon nutmeg
1 tablespoon white miso
½ cup raw cashew butter
chopped parsley for garnish

Steam cauliflower and garlic in a steamer for about 15 minutes or until tender. In a large skillet, steam-sauté the leeks and red bell pepper about 8 to 10 minutes until soft. Add mushrooms and steam-sauté for another 2 minutes until mushrooms soften. Mix in nutmeg and white miso. Transfer cauliflower and garlic to a mixing bowl. Mash cauliflower, garlic, and cashew butter with potato masher or fork. Gently stir in leek mixture. Serve sprinkled with fresh parsley.

VEGETABLE MASHED SWEET POTATOES
Servings: 6

4 large sweet potatoes
5 cloves garlic, pressed
2 medium zucchini, grated
1 pound fresh washed spinach
    (baby, shredded, or cooked frozen)
2 teaspoons Bragg Liquid Amino
    Acids
¼ teaspoon nutmeg

Bake or microwave sweet potatoes until soft. Peel and mash in bowl. Microwave garlic, zucchini, and spinach about 1 to 2 minutes until spinach is just wilted. Turn vegetables into bowl with mashed sweet potatoes. Add Bragg and nutmeg and mix all ingredients together.

STOVETOP RATATOUILLE
Servings: 4

6 medium zucchini, cut in ½-inch
    rounds
1 large eggplant, cut in 1-inch
    cubes (if organic, do not peel)
1 onion, chopped
6 cloves garlic, minced or pressed
1 (28-ounce) can crushed
    tomatoes, no salt
1 pound mushrooms, sliced
2 teaspoons chopped fresh thyme
    or 1 teaspoon dried
1 teaspoon chopped fresh rosemary
    or ½ teaspoon dried

In large saucepan, cover and slowly simmer all ingredients, stirring occasionally, for 15 to 20 minutes or until tender. The tomatoes and vegetables will make their own sauce.

AUTUMN HARVEST STUFFED WINTER SQUASH
Servings: 2

1 winter squash, cut in half and
    seeds removed
2 tablespoons chopped dried
    apricots
2 tablespoons dried currants
½ cup frozen cherries, defrosted
2 tablespoons chopped raw walnuts
powdered cinnamon

Preheat oven to 350 degrees. Bake squash facedown in ½-inch of water for 45 minutes. Mix dried fruit, cherries, and nuts. When squash is tender, fill cavity with fruit and nut mixture. Sprinkle with cinnamon and bake for an additional 30 minutes.

CREAMY KALE WITH MUSHROOMS AND ONIONS
Servings: 6

2 bunches kale
1 large onion, coarsely chopped
8 cloves garlic, sliced
½ pound shiitake mushrooms, sliced
½ pound white mushrooms, sliced
3 tablespoons dried currants
3 tablespoons raw cashew or almond butter
2 teaspoons white miso
1 tablespoon balsamic vinegar

Remove the thick bottom of the stems from the kale and coarsely chop. Steam-sauté kale, onion, and garlic for 10 minutes until tender. Add mushrooms and steam-sauté for another 5 minutes. Add the rest of the ingredients and toss well.

Note: To make a complete meal, add cooked or canned beans at the end and heat through.

STEAMED BROCCOLI AND RED BELL PEPPER WITH OLIVE OIL AND GARLIC
Servings: 4

1 bunch broccoli, cut into small florets
1 red bell pepper, seeded and thinly sliced
6 cloves garlic, peeled and sliced lengthwise
3 teaspoons cold-pressed virgin olive oil

Steam broccoli, bell pepper, and garlic until broccoli is just tender, about 7 to 10 minutes. Drizzle with olive oil and serve.

ROASTED FENNEL
Servings: 4

2 large fennel bulbs, green stalk removed and root end trimmed (save a few fennel sprigs)
2 teaspoons cold-pressed olive oil
3 cloves garlic, pressed
1 lemon or lime, cut in half

heat the oven to 375
...s. Wash the trimmed fennel
bulb well. Stand it on a cutting
board in a vertical position and cut
into ½-inch slices. In a shallow
baking dish, toss the fennel with
olive oil and garlic and arrange
slices in a single layer. Roast the
fennel for 15 to 20 minutes, and
turn carefully to brown the other
side. When tender and browned, 35
to 40 minutes, remove from oven
and squeeze lemon or lime over it.
Garnish the dish with the delicate
fennel sprigs.

LEMONY GREEN BEANS
AND PINE NUTS
Servings: 6

1½ pounds green beans, trimmed
    and cut diagonally into ½-inch
    pieces
¼ cup pine nuts, lightly toasted
2 tablespoons finely chopped parsley
1½ teaspoons organic lemon zest
3 teaspoons cold-pressed olive oil
2 teaspoons Bragg Liquid Amino
    Acids

Steam beans until just tender,
about 5 minutes. Transfer to a bowl
and toss with the rest of the ingredients.

SWEET-AND-SOUR RED CABBAGE
WITH BLUEBERRIES AND FENNEL
Servings: 4

3½ cups thinly sliced red cabbage
1 medium fennel bulb (sometimes
    called anise), stalks trimmed
    flush with bulb and bulb
    chopped fine
½ cup water
¼ cup cider vinegar
4 tablespoons dehydrated date
    sugar (found in health food
    stores)
1 teaspoon Bragg Liquid Amino
    Acids
1 cup fresh or frozen blueberries
1 teaspoon cold-pressed olive oil

In a large heavy nonstick skillet,
steam-sauté cabbage over moderate
heat, stirring and adding water as
necessary, until wilted slightly,
about 5 to 10 minutes. Add fennel
and cook, stirring, until just tender,
about 5 minutes. Stir in water,
vinegar, and date sugar, and cook
over moderately low heat, covered.
Stir occasionally, until vegetables
are tender and liquid is almost
evaporated, 10 or 15 minutes. Add
blueberries and heat until hot. Toss
in oil. Serve hot or at room temperature.

BROCCOLI WITH CURRANTS AND PINE NUTS
Servings: 4

¼ cup pine nuts
1 head broccoli, florets
3 garlic cloves, minced or pressed
⅓ cup dry sherry or white wine
¼ cup currants or raisins
½ teaspoon crushed red pepper
2 teaspoons Bragg Liquid Amino Acids
2 teaspoons cold-pressed olive oil

In extra-large skillet over medium heat, carefully dry-roast pine nuts, stirring constantly, until fragrant and just barely golden, 1 to 2 minutes. Add broccoli, garlic, sherry, currants, and crushed red pepper and cover pan. Cook, stirring occasionally, until broccoli is tender, 7 to 10 minutes. Toss with Bragg and olive oil and serve.

Note: Pecans, walnuts, or hazelnuts can be substituted for the pine nuts.

DESSERTS

TROPICAL FRUIT COMPOTE
Servings: 6

1 cup cubed mango
2 cups cubed pineapple

2 oranges, peeled, sliced, and seeded
1 sliced banana
1 cup cubed papaya
2 tablespoons unsweetened shredded coconut (optional)

Toss together and serve.

SIMPLE CHOCOLATE-NUT DIP FOR FRUIT AND STRAWBERRIES
Servings: 10

1 cup raw macadamia nuts, raw cashews, or blanched almonds, unsalted
1 teaspoon vanilla extract
2 tablespoons cocoa powder
⅔ cup pitted dates
1 cup soy milk

In blender or food processor, blend ingredients together until smooth and creamy. In blender, you may need to add more soy milk, and stop and stir occasionally until smooth.

Note: For a vanilla dip, omit the cocoa powder.

CREAMY FRUIT COMPOTE
Servings: 10

2 large organic apples, sweet, tart, and crisp, cut in bite-sized cubes

1 pint fresh strawberries

4 kiwis, peeled and cut

2 oranges, peeled past skin, sliced in rounds, and seeded

1 pineapple, cored, peeled, and cut in bite-sized chunks

2 cups halved grapes

¼ cup unsweetened shredded coconut meat (found in health food stores)

½ cup unsweetened dried cherries, or cranberries or raisins (optional)

⅔ cup chopped walnuts or pecans

Citrus-Cashew Dressing

2 oranges, peeled and seeded

2 tablespoons rice vinegar

½ cup raw cashews

½ cup goji berries (optional)

orange juice

In a blender, combine dressing ingredients and blend until smooth and creamy. Add orange juice to thin if necessary. Toss apples in a little orange juice to prevent browning. Combine all ingredients, using only ½ cup of the walnuts, right before serving. Toss with dressing and garnish with the remaining walnuts.

Note: Great for a holiday feast.

POMEGRANATE POACHED PEARS WITH BERRY-BERRY SAUCE
Servings: 6

Poached Pears

6 medium pears, ripe but still firm

2 cups unsweetened pomegranate juice

1 whole cinnamon stick

6 whole cloves

goji berries for garnish

fresh blueberries for garnish

Berry-Berry Sauce

⅔ cup raw cashews, unsalted

½ cup frozen strawberries, defrosted

1 cup frozen blueberries, defrosted

8 pitted dates

1 cup soy milk

Peel pears, leaving stems intact. Slice a little off the bottom of each pear so they stand up. In a large saucepan, place pears standing up snugly together. Pour in pomegranate juice and add cinnamon stick and cloves. Gently simmer, covered, for about 15 to 20 minutes until pears are tender. Gently remove pears and refrigerate until ready to serve. Reduce poaching liquid over high heat until it becomes syrup. Chill syrup until serving.

In blender or food processor, blend together all sauce ingredients for 2 to 3 minutes until very smooth and creamy.

To serve, place pear on dessert plate and pour pomegranate syrup over pear, followed by Berry-Berry Sauce. Sprinkle a few fresh blueberries on plate and top pears with a sprinkle of red goji berries for a sight to behold.

Note: Tastes so decadent, but it is really healthy and guilt-free!!

CHOCOLATE JUBILEE PUDDING CAKE
Servings: 12

Cake

1⅔ cups spelt flour
3 teaspoons baking soda
1 teaspoon baking powder
3 cups pitted dates
1 cup frozen cherries, thawed
½ cup prunes
1 whole banana
2 cups unsweetened applesauce
1 cup shredded beets
¾ cup shredded carrots
½ cup shredded zucchini
1½ cups water
1 cup chopped walnuts
½ cup unsweetened shredded coconut, rehydrated with ½ cup water
½ cup currants
½ cup sliced pitted dates
3 tablespoons cocoa powder— natural, not Dutch processed
2 teaspoons vanilla extract

Chocolate-Cherry Nut Topping

½ cup raw macadamia nuts, unsalted
½ cup raw cashew nuts
½ cup frozen cherries, thawed
3 tablespoons cocoa powder
1 teaspoon vanilla extract
⅔ cup pitted dates
⅔ cup soy milk

Preheat oven to 350 degrees. Mix flour, baking powder, and baking soda in a bowl. In blender, blend 3 cups dates, cherries, prunes, banana, and applesauce together. In large bowl, mix beets, carrots, zucchini, water, blended mixture, walnuts, coconut, currants, sliced dates, cocoa powder, and vanilla. Add the flour mixture. Mix well and spread in a nonstick 9x13-inch cake pan. Bake for about 1 hour or until a toothpick inserted into the center comes out clean.

In powerful blender or food processor, blend together topping ingredients until smooth and creamy. In food processor, the icing will not become as smooth and creamy. Place a dollop over warm cake and serve.

STRAWBERRY SAUCE
Servings: 8–10

½ cup vanilla soy milk
¼ cup cashew nuts
½ bag frozen strawberries, thawed
1 tablespoon date sugar, or 2 dates

Blend all ingredients together and serve over fruit salad, poached pears, or Baked Fruit Delight.

BAKED FRUIT DELIGHT
Servings: 10

6 Granny Smith apples, peeled and
   sliced
8 dates, pitted and chopped
1 cup goji berries or currants
1 cup frozen cherries
1 cup frozen blueberries
1 cup crushed pineapple with juice
¼ cup water
¾ cup chopped walnuts or pecans
½ teaspoon cinnamon
¼ teaspoon nutmeg
juice of 1 orange
2 teaspoons organic lemon zest

Preheat oven to 350 degrees. Mix all ingredients. Put in a cov-

ered pan and bake 30 minutes or until soft.

Note: Great served warm with cold strawberry sauce or topped with Robin's Very Berry Creamy Ice Cream.

ROBIN'S VERY BERRY
CREAMY ICE CREAM
Servings: 6–8

2 cups soy milk
⅔ cup raw cashews
12 pitted dates
1½ cups frozen blueberries
1½ cups frozen strawberries

Blend thoroughly in a blender and freeze in an ice cream maker.

CHOCOLATE DIVINE
MOUSSE ICE CREAM
Servings: 6–8

2 cups soy milk
⅔ cup soft tofu
⅔ cup raw cashews
16 pitted dates
2 handfuls fresh baby spinach
   (exact quantity not critical)
1 cup frozen blueberries
1 cup frozen unsweetened cherries
3 heaping tablespoons of natural
   (not Dutch processed) cocoa

2 tablespoons flaxseed
1 teaspoon vanilla
1 tablespoon Kahlua (optional)

Mix thoroughly in a blender for several minutes until smooth and silky and then freeze in an ice cream maker.

Note: You can also just mix this up, keep it in the refrigerator, and eat it as pudding. That was one five-year-old's idea.

PART III

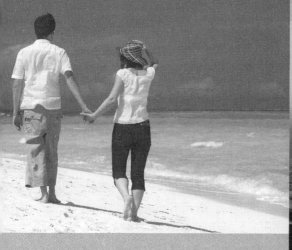

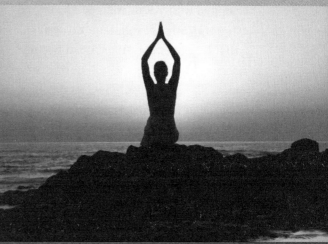

JOURNEY TO WHOLENESS

The most beautiful and profound emotion we
can experience is the sensation of the mysterious.
It is the power of all true science.

—Albert Einstein

INTRODUCTION

With food, we feed our outer bodies. With wisdom, we feed our souls.

What defines happiness? Is it success, achievement, or a comfortable space in life? I thought I'd found happiness when I became a princess. No, I was not born into nobility. I married a prince.

In my early twenties, I left home to fulfill my dream of happiness. I was equipped with youth and good looks, an extremely strong will, but no realistic goals. By age twenty-two, I had become a princess with access to a country castle and a villa in Vienna. This should have been the pinnacle of my life, right?

It took less than a year to realize that happiness comes from within, not from others. As I spent my days thinking of new ways to experience my social status, I began focusing on my looks and worrying about how people viewed me. I didn't feel popular or accepted.

I recall one event that made me realize the extent of my true unhappiness. My husband and I were staying at my in-laws' castle. It was an enchanting setting—elegant furniture, lovely gardens, near a charming village and the Danube River. I hardly noticed it. I was too busy complaining to my husband about the behavior of others.

One night we argued, and I escaped to the salon (living room). I was pouting, depressed, and feeling very sorry for myself. Suddenly, I began looking around at the luxury surrounding me. The room was quiet and peaceful. The moon was full and its soft rays shone through the French doors.

Suddenly, I realized that as a princess I was miserable. I had put all my energy into external achievements and possessions without finding happiness. I didn't even know how to define it anymore. I just knew I didn't have it. From that day on, I began searching for spiritual wisdom instead of chasing after happiness.

Years later, I had an unbelievable experience—a tragic horseback-riding accident. What happened that day pushed me to an even higher level of spiritual insight, truth, and wisdom. I also realized that finding wisdom and truth is a lifelong process.

About two years after the accident, I was living on Grand Cayman Island and working as a private chef for a wealthy couple. I enjoyed the freshest and highest quality of foods. Because I focused on nutrition as a chef, I ate and prepared only nutritious foods. My way of eating gave me mental and spiritual clarity and my health dramatically improved. I was also exposed to the vast wisdom my employer shared with me on a daily basis.

Most mornings, I would walk through the plush Eden-like grounds of a five-star hotel en route to a charming little café. At the café, I would read while sipping tea. One day, while engrossed in a spiritual book, I was motivated to ask God to help me understand the book's message. I bowed my head briefly in silent prayer.

Upon opening my eyes, I saw a couple of obese people eating pastries. As I looked around the café, I saw that *everyone* was eating this way. Then I noticed the expressions on their faces—frustration, dissatisfaction, fret, worry . . .

What is going on here? I wondered. *Most of these people are on vacation in this paradise, yet they appear miserable.*

Walking back through the hotel grounds, I noticed that a manmade stream looked fake and contrived. Then I glanced over at a statue I'd passed by many times. I stopped in my tracks and I suddenly noticed just how disgusting it was. It had a grotesque and grimacing face, horns on its head, and writhing snakelike creatures slithering out of its orifices. I stopped an employee and asked him to look at the statue and tell me what he saw. He, too, saw a hideous form. We couldn't imagine why the hotel would put such an ugly statue on its grounds.

Next I noticed a well-dressed couple that appeared disgruntled and upset with each other. The bleary-eyed man looked like he'd had way too much to drink the night before. *Why were they so miserable?*

A few days later, I was sitting on the patio of a charming beachside restaurant when I noticed a group of black birds stealing scraps of food from the tables and floor. At first, the birds' antics amused me, but they began flocking around the artificial sweetener packets from an empty table. They ignored the sugar packets but frantically tore open the sweetener packets as if gorging on cocaine. These birds seemed addicted, and with their black beaks coated in powder, they began feeding the "drug" to the younger birds.

As I sat watching the birds and recalling the other events that had caught my attention, my eyes began to open. We are part of a very influential and powerful world. Often unknowingly, we accept cultural norms that influence our actions and behaviors in negative ways. We long to fit in, for better or worse, even if it may harm us.

Optimal health is much more than *physical* health. We must be willing to *open our eyes* to receive it. When we live against the way we were designed to live, we live in a state of unhappiness. We can't simply desire to see the truth, we must have the power to act upon our wisdom.

After my serious horseback-riding accident, I vowed to do whatever was necessary to stay healthy and out of the hospital. By making that vow, I was asking the Creator to show me a way. I immersed myself in both the Old and New Testaments of the Bible. I had always viewed the Old Testament as a laundry list of "begets" and "commandments." But *with my new eyes*, I began focusing on the Pentateuch or written Torah, the first five books of the Bible. I quickly recognized the practical life instruction that the Torah provides.

I am not formally trained as a scientist, theologian, or psychologist. I am just a person who has overcome many obstacles and learned by observing my own behavior and the behaviors of others. Most importantly, I believe in a God of love, mercy, and forgiveness. I feel my Creator has called me to share these enlightening experiences and knowledge with you.

JOURNEY TO WHOLENESS

When we are relaxed, we provide our cells with sufficient nutrients and energy to feed our organs. During times of stress or threat, the energy we normally

use for logical reasoning and organ function is diverted.

We've all been in stressful situations where we didn't think clearly or react normally. We might have said things or behaved totally out of character. We are designed to cope with stress temporarily—long enough to deal with the threat—and then we return to a relaxed state, *right?* Unfortunately, this fast-paced world keeps us locked up in a stressful, messy state.

While the Super Antioxidant Diet provides the tools for achieving health on a cellular level, the Journey to Wholeness section provides the tools for transforming psychological and spiritual states to a place of calmness, awareness, and resiliency. By addressing the whole person—body, mind, and spirit—you can fully experience the journey toward optimal health.

This section includes the following chapters:

Emotions • Thoughts
Relaxation • Inner Voices
Awareness • Forgiveness
Nurturing • Attitude
Social Pressure

The exercises included in this section are not always easy. In fact, I recommend that you do each exercise for at least a week before moving on to the next one. You might want to repeat the exercises at a later time, as they will help you grow in awareness at a more receptive time in your life.

I also recommend that you incorporate the exercises from the Inner Voices and Relaxation chapters into your daily life. By taking the time to regularly practice these exercises while following the diet plan, you will develop:

- Increased conscious awareness of yourself, others, and your overall environment

- Increased ability to focus

- Ability to harness your mind

- Increased spiritual awareness

- Increased ability to make better choices

Each of the exercises in this section introduces the simplest aspects of several ancient disciplines. You may choose to learn more about all or any one of these disciplines as you learn to follow your individual path toward optimal health.

CHAPTER FIFTEEN

EMOTIONS

Emotions are very powerful, and we all struggle to interpret them. They influence our decisions, our moods, and our interactions with others. When negative emotions become the "norm," our reaction to them often becomes a habit. Instead of looking for the source, many people simply learn how to cope by developing habits of escape—habits like overeating, heavy drinking, risky sex, overspending, or becoming addicted to medication. Others throw themselves into their work and become obsessed with making money or gaining power. Still others become obsessed with their appearance. Some people just give up.

We've all felt the heaviness of stress, of feeling out of control.

Why do we do the things we do? Is it possible we have become disconnected from our spiritual origin and how we were meant to live? My personal life change resulted from an encounter with my Creator, a diet rich in antioxidant foods, and an active decision to focus on positive thoughts and actions. I have also spent years researching the Bible in its original languages. In addition, I have continually sought out books, articles, and studies related to psychology, spirituality, and neuroscience.

People who change old patterns can actually change how their cells and bodies react. In other words, we can actually transform ourselves by resetting the way we think and feel. Practicing positive thinking is just as important as practicing healthy eating.

Accept that we live in a world where pleasure has become a goal. Just look at the media. It is *all about* "feeling good." After all, "feeling good" is what sells. No wonder 99 percent of the population feels worthless and unimportant. But even the media-makers have personal lives that reflect dissatisfaction and depression. In reality, we are all the same.

As a professional chef, I have worked with wealthy celebrities and non-celebrities. They share the same insecurities and fears we do—maybe even more so as they are forced to live up to the expectations in the glare of the public lens. Life is just not easy for any of us.

We must accept that the world we see in the media is not real, and pleasurable emotions cannot be ongoing. If we always felt good, how would we know it, with nothing in our lives with which to compare it?

Become aware of your feelings. When we are young, we learn from our interactions and surroundings. In a perfect world, our role models and parents would reflect perfect life skills, and school friends or siblings would always be kind and respectful. How idealistic!

As we grow up, we form our own habits of coping. Our true feelings often become hardened or ignored because of painful, negative reminders.

Remember that childhood game of hot/cold—in which someone is given clues to something's location by saying warm (meaning nearby), hot (almost on top of it), and cool/cold (the opposite). It's funny, but the hot/cold game can actually help in the journey toward emotional wholeness.

Having a quiet, peaceful experience is a good indicator that we are going the right way. Feeling uncomfortable is an indicator that something is not right.

Emotions can serve as guideposts or markers. Accept and identify these feelings.

Realize that the consequences of making bad choices may result in unpleasant emotions. You've heard people say, "I just feel numb." Yes, because many negative events and emotions result from our unwise choices, not as cruel punishment. The emotions from numerous negative events accumulate and often cause depression and numbness. The purpose of negative emotions is to motivate change and improve the ability to make wiser choices. Wise choices also reward with a sense of integrity and clarity. Being open to doing things more positively, which may sometimes feel very unfamiliar and uncomfortable, will help us achieve a more fulfilling life.

Some people become inundated with painful emotions, and never recognize the emotional guideposts as a way out of the maze. Instead, they run away, adding to the vicious cycle of more unwise choices.

Choosing the quick fix may appear easier, but nothing could be further from the truth. Over time, quick-fix consequences often create disastrous results. Some dietary and sedentary lifestyle consequences are obesity, high blood pressure, cancer, heart attacks, feelings of guilt, condemnation, or anger, and mental degeneration.

Recognize that change takes time and practice. For thousands of years, ancient spiritual disciplines have recognized the need to slow down and appreciate life more fully—to actually experience the body and all of the sensations, pleasant and unpleasant.

Recent studies in neuroscience, quantum physics, and cellular biology are revealing that people can actually create health and well-being by rewiring their brains through the power of choice. You are not a victim of your genes or your environment; you can change the course of your life!

Research scientist Bruce Lipton, PhD, states in his book *The Biology of Belief:*[1]

The implications of this research radically change our understanding of life. It shows that genes and DNA do not control our biology; that instead DNA is controlled by signals from outside the cell, including the energetic messages emanating from our positive and negative thoughts. . . .

This profoundly hopeful synthesis of the latest and best research in cell biology and quantum physics is being hailed as a major breakthrough, showing that our bodies can be changed as we retrain our thinking.

Whether we like it or not, we are wired to respond to a simple reward/discipline system. How much simpler could it be? Understanding this concept is one of the clues to keeping on the straight path and out of the mazes.

This world is complex and confusing; people are overwhelmed by a flood of choices and, more often than not, unhealthy choices. Denial has become a common mode of escape. It anesthetizes people and keeps them trapped in a vicious maze. Decisions are made from a sort of autopilot state. This is extremely frustrating because even though we know we are making harmful choices, we continue to do so over and over again.

EXERCISE: EMOTIONAL CHECKUP

Keep a record of your emotions in a pocket journal designated just for exercises. I recommend you practice *this* exercise for six weeks while following one of our meal plans. In this way, you will have enough time to experience remarkable results from your new eating pattern, which will increase your motivation to continue.

Record the time, date, and emotion(s) you are feeling when:

• First awake

• Before you eat or drink anything

• Before going to bed.

The following list of emotions, though certainly not all-inclusive, can help you get started:

Happy • Angry • Offended
Sad • Guilty • Excited
Anxious • Ashamed • Euphoric
Scared • Frustrated • Hyper
Secure • Disorganized
Peaceful • Irritated
Confused • Bored

As you record each day, you may be surprised by some of the emotions you experience. You may even make some helpful connections. At this phase, just observe your emotions, don't judge them. Remember, becoming aware helps you attain wisdom!

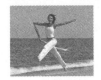

CHAPTER SIXTEEN

THOUGHTS

As a man thinketh in his heart so he is.
—Proverbs 23:7

Underlying thoughts are behind every mood, feeling, and emotion. Thoughts, both negative and positive, release powerful brain chemicals that signal us to react in certain ways. By becoming consciously aware of our thoughts, we are able to identify the triggers that result in certain responses and behaviors. A trigger for overeating, for instance, may result from feelings of helplessness, depression, or powerlessness.

In the first exercise, you became more aware of the emotions you experience throughout the day. In this exercise, you will list the thoughts and behaviors associated with the emotions you feel at those different times of the day.

EXERCISE: IDENTIFYING YOUR THOUGHTS

When you wake up each morning, before you eat or drink, and before you retire at night, record:

- Feelings

- Thought reactions

- Possible solutions

No matter how absurd these thoughts may seem, write them down! At the end of the evening, look over your daily journal and ask yourself these three questions:

1. What were the emotions?

2. What were the thoughts associated with the emotions?

3. What solutions did I create as a result of these emotions and thoughts?

You may be wondering what this has to do with your overall health. Hold on. You will soon understand.

CHAPTER SEVENTEEN

RELAXATION

Our response to thoughts, emotions, and experiences affects our ability to breathe, relax, and sleep. Correct breathing helps us to relax and regain a sense of calmness.

BREATHING

Breathing is inseparable from consciousness and health. The deep and free-flowing breath we enjoy when relaxed becomes jerky and short when we experience stress and discomfort. When stress and discomfort become natural states, shallow breathing becomes a habit and can suck the spirit right out of us.

Correct Breathing

• Increases absorption of nutrients

• Maintains optimal cellular oxygenation, which helps the body maintain an ideal pH

• Expels cellular toxins that cause weight-regulating glands to be sluggish

• More than doubles the amount of body fat that is oxidized and burned

Our breathing is a reaction to our environment and creates resulting thoughts. By observing our breath, we become aware of what's really happening inside us. Think of your breath as the constant ebb and flow of ocean tides.

A friend told me about a ten-day meditation course that involves the focused awareness of breathing. One of the steps in overcoming mental garbage is to focus on the breath.

In *The Breathing Book*, author Donna Farhi states: "Full body breathing is an extraordinary symphony of both powerful and subtle movements that massage our internal organs, oscillate our joints, and alternately tone and release all the muscles in the body."[1]

We are taught to stand up straight and suck in our stomachs. Constantly holding the stomach in causes muscles to weaken. You must relax and contract muscles in order to strengthen them. After all, you don't see weight lifters just holding weights in the air, do you? They must contract and relax their muscles in order to build strength.

As a person keeps the stomach in constant contraction, breathing is constricted to the chest area. Chest breathing alerts the brain to prepare for a stressful situation. In other words, breathing from the chest keeps us in a state of anxiety. Breathing from the belly induces the production of relaxing brain chemicals.

At a primal level, we are designed to breathe from our abdomens when there is no threat of danger, so we can relax. In other words, breathing from the belly is a natural tranquilizer! Keeping the bloodstream oxygenated also lowers the production of stress hormones.

In today's chronically stressful culture, the body isn't often given the opportunity to repair itself. The secretion of the hormone cortisol into the bloodstream is one response to stress. Cortisol has been dubbed the "stress hormone." According to studies, the overproduction of the hormone cortisol may contribute to food bingeing.[2,3]

Caffeine, refined sugars (anything not from whole fruit), and an excess of starchy foods (especially refined carbohydrates such as white flour and white rice) also raise cortisol levels. Dr. Nicholas Perricone reports: "A study conducted at Duke University found that the effects of morning coffee consumption can exaggerate the body's stress responses and increase stress hormone levels all day long and into the evening. This is a high price to pay for that morning jolt to our systems."[4]

Chronic stress, with higher and prolonged levels of cortisol in the bloodstream, has been shown to have the following negative effects:

- Impaired cognitive performance

- Suppressed thyroid function

- Blood sugar imbalances such as hypoglycemia

- Decreased bone density

- Decrease in muscle tissue

- Higher blood pressure

- Lowered immunity

- Inflammatory responses in the body (after a time this causes inflammatory diseases—diseases that end in the suffix "itis," such as arthritis)

- Increased abdominal fat

Proper belly breathing has been found by many to be very helpful in relaxing the body and mind—thus maintaining healthy cortisol levels.

You can do this next exercise anywhere at any time. I suggest that you wear loose clothing so you might better focus on your breathing.

EXERCISE ONE: FOCUS ON BREATHING

Step One

Evaluate your breathing by asking these questions:

- Does my breath originate in my nostrils, chest, or abdomen? Does it feel shortened?

- Is my breath smooth and flowing or labored, jerky, short, rhythmic, and mechanical?

- Do I pause after I exhale?

- Do I inhale through my nose or mouth? Do I exhale through my nose or mouth?

- What am I thinking or feeling as I breathe?

As you become more aware of your breathing, you will allow it to become smoother.

Step Two

Repeat Step One until you are fully aware of your breathing patterns.

Step Three

- Lie down on your back and relax.

- Place your hand on your belly.

- Focus on breathing through your nose, past your chest, and into your abdomen. Your belly will rise.

- You may exhale through your nose or mouth. Your belly will fall as you exhale.

- Practice this until you get the hang of it.

EXERCISE TWO: "THE BEACH"

"The Beach" is a breathing/relaxation exercise a friend of mine shared with her son to help him go to sleep at night. He continues to use it to this day! With practice, you will be able to "feel" the relaxing images in your mind.

Step One

Lie down in a quiet, dimly lit, comfortable place. Close your eyes and imagine you are on a beach. Repeat these thoughts to yourself:

- I am lying on a beach. I am relaxed and motionless. (Pause and focus on taking deep breaths.)

- I feel the warm sand soothing my back.

- I feel the warmth of the lazy sun on my skin. (Pause and focus on taking deep breaths.)

- I hear the quiet waves pulsating and feel the cool water touching my skin. (Pause and focus on taking deep breaths.)

- I smell the clean ocean air. I feel a cool breeze across my skin.

- I am relaxed and motionless. (Pause and focus on taking deep breaths.)

Step Two

Repeat Step One.

Step Three

Relax your muscles from head to toe. Repeat these thoughts:

- I feel the muscles in the top of my head relaxing. (Pause to relax.)

- I feel my ears relaxing. (Pause to relax the ears.)

- I feel the muscles in my eyes and forehead relax. (Pause to relax the eyes and forehead. Focus on taking deep breaths.)

- Continue this until you have relaxed the muscles of the face, the neck, the base of the neck, the shoulders, the top of the arms, the forearms, the hands to the tip of each finger, the top of the back, the middle of the back, the lower back, the chest, the lungs, the buttocks, the thighs, the calves, the feet, and the toes.

Step Four

Repeat "I am relaxed and motionless." (Pause and focus on deep breaths each time.)

Whatever exercise you use to relax or sleep, focus on breathing from the belly. Every time you check in with your breathing, remind yourself to belly breathe. You will notice how relaxed and calm you become. By changing your breath, you might experience some unusual emotions that have been repressed due to your chest breathing.

Just observe the emotions, allow them to come forth, and keep breathing naturally from your belly. This is an essential lifetime habit for health.

ADEQUATE RELAXATION

Abstain from any sort of work one day a week. Just relax and enjoy the day. I decided to rest on Saturday, the seventh day of the week. When I began keeping Sabbath from Friday sunset to Saturday sunset, my system began to quiet down.

There have been times when I have chosen to work a seven-day week, working on the Sabbath, but each time I was tired and less efficient the following week.

CHAPTER EIGHTEEN

INNER VOICES

Have you ever gotten lost but eventually found your way? Have you ever sensed danger or caution without really knowing why?

I recently read about this "sixth sense" phenomenon in Malcolm Gladwell's best-selling book, *Blink*.[1] He writes about a Greek statue dating from the sixth century B.C.E. A Getty Museum curator was given the task of authenticating the piece prior to the museum purchasing it.

The curator proudly unveiled the statue for several experts and each one had an immediate reaction. One expert heard the word "fresh" in his mind, another experienced an unexplainable repulsion, and another expert couldn't take her eyes off the statue's fingernails. Something just didn't seem right! Each expert shared the sudden reaction that the statue was fake.

The preliminary scientific evidence refuted the experts' "gut feelings."

Nonetheless, the purchase was postponed so the statue could be subjected to more rigorous testing. The statue was indeed an excellent fraud.

How did those experts "know" without any proof that something was not right? I believe it was that still, small voice of truth that we all experience. Some refer to it as intuition, a hunch, or a gut feeling, while others believe it to be the inner voice of God or Spirit.

Why do we have this feeling from time to time? Or do you choose to ignore it in this busy, stressful world? Do you *ask* to hear it? Do you ask to know? Matthew 7:7–8 says: *"Seek and you shall find. Ask and you shall receive."* If we don't ask, we will never reveal a sense of knowing. Think about that.

In this section, you will learn how to turn off the business of life and experience conscious awareness.

As you begin watching your thoughts, you will experience mental chatter. The mind chatter is agitating and will probably make you squirm. It may take on the voice or attitude of a parent, a significant other, a sibling, or even you. You may get emotional.

With practice, you will learn how to overcome this mind chatter and experience the voice of "quiet."

EXERCISE ONE: LISTENING TO HEAR

Step One

Pick a time each day, preferably early morning or before you sleep, to be alone for at least twenty minutes. It doesn't really matter *where* you are, as long as you can get away from daily distractions. After you have practiced and are comfortable with Step One, go on to Step Two. When you are comfortable with Step Two, go on to Step Three. Record each experience in your journal.

- Sit in a comfortable position on a soft surface such as a pillow.

- Relax your entire body. Close your eyes. Place the palms of your hands together in a relaxed cupping position.

- Focus on taking deep breaths.

- Place your internal gaze on the back of your forehead as if it were the wall of a cave. Listen to your surroundings and feel your body. Don't strain your eyes.

- Be aware of the tips of your fingers touching each other. Notice each finger. (Pause and focus on taking deep breaths.)

- Allow your thoughts to pass by like a train. Observe them without judgment.

- Relax your body if it tenses.

- Gently bring your awareness back to your hands and settle your internal gaze on the wall inside your forehead.

- Allow your mind to hear and your body to feel each breath.

- If you experience distractions, bring your awareness back to your hands and the back of your forehead.

- When finished, open your eyes and become aware of your surroundings.

Step Two

Before going to bed, begin with Step One. After observing your breath, your hands, and your forehead:

• Allow the events of the day to surface.

• Observe each uncomfortable event, such as:

  • Any misjudgment of or negativity toward you.

  • Any judgment or negative thought you had toward someone else.

• Acknowledge each negative thought. If you took part in an unkind thought or deed, acknowledge it, receive forgiveness, and release. If you were the recipient of an unkind thought or deed, acknowledge it, forgive, and release.

• Once completed, return your awareness to your breath, your hands, and your forehead.

Step Three

When we release worldly, negative thoughts, our beings become clear and focused. Now, it is time for you to experience self-forgiveness, inspiration, and positive thinking. Begin this step by completing the first two steps, then:

• Remind yourself there is no yesterday or tomorrow, only an instance of the present.

• Acknowledge your gifts and strengths.

• Let go of all negative chatter.

• Release all negativity.

• Record all present and future thoughts, ideas, reminders, and instructions as they flow into your mind.

• Remind yourself that you are part of the "bigger whole" of humanity.

DIFFICULT PEOPLE

People that irritate us often come into our lives, but every interaction happens for a reason. Perhaps this person is a demanding boss, a chatterbox coworker, an intrusive drunk on a plane.

One time, I was at the gym and the older man exercising next to me began rasping and clearing his throat like he had a chest cold. *How dare he come to the gym with a cold*, I thought. I "humphed" several times to get his attention but finally asked in an intolerant voice, "Are you sick or something?"

He looked over at me and apologized. "No, I have asthma and exercise does help me a great deal. I hope I'm not too loud."

I felt horrible about my negative judgment of him. Now when I see him at the gym, we talk about family and life. I don't even notice his rasping anymore. This experience made me think about what I might be doing that irritates those around me. We are all reflections of each other, after all!

CHAPTER NINETEEN

AWARENESS

If you have followed the guides and exercises in this book, you most certainly are beginning to experience a transformation process. You have experienced either great relief or tribulation. Each experience will proceed at its own pace. Remember to focus on each day and know that you will eventually experience balance.

Most people live in an emotional "now" world rather than the mental "see the big picture" world. Those who have conquered the emotional world often go on to achieve great things. We hear about them in the news. They are what we term the "driven" ones: the cutting-edge scientists, established authors, phenomenal athletes, social activists, creative artists and musicians, the innovative entrepreneurs, and so on.

Bookstores are full of self-help books and motivational programs that promise the keys to accomplishment. Wealth, power, and success are meaningless if accomplished without balance and awareness.

EXERCISE ONE: EXPERIENCING AWARENESS

Whether you are an emotional world person or mental world person, this exercise has been designed to help you become more aware of your surroundings and body.

Pick a physical activity that you think you would enjoy. Walking is a great time to connect with your environment, process your thoughts, enjoy the company of a friend, or get to know your children. I love to walk through the wooded areas near my house. You may enjoy exercising at a health club, participating in group sports, dancing, horseback riding, swimming, or running. The key is to find what you like and be completely aware of the physical experience surrounding the activity.

Remember "The Beach" exercise in which you experienced your senses of the imagined water, air, and sounds? Now you will experience your senses in the physical world. You can do this exercise during any activity, like walking down the street, for instance.

As you walk down the street, notice the leaves shimmering in the breeze. Feel the breeze on your face and body. Listen to the sound of your footsteps. Become aware of the warmth of the sun, the chirping of birds, your breaths, and other sounds around you. What are the colors you see? What smells fill the air?

While driving your car, feel the steering wheel, listen to the sounds, breath in and notice the scents, observe your thoughts, feel your foot on the gas pedal, observe your surroundings and the cars around you.

As thoughts pop into your mind, shift your focus to how your body is experiencing the environment. Simply experience yourself in your body. Is it a pleasant experience? The more pleasant experiences you create, the better your mind functions. *Just become aware of the present.*

EXERCISE TWO: FOOD AWARENESS

This exercise will help you to appreciate the subtle qualities of food as well as become present to consciously experiencing and enjoying the food you eat.

Place different vegetables, fruits, and nuts in front of you. Completely focus on each item. Look at its details, feel it, smell it, taste it, notice its texture in your mouth as you slowly chew it. Is it sweet, bitter, salty, or sour? Notice the subtle flavors. Notice the water content, dryness, or oiliness of the food.

What are your thoughts about the food? Think about how you are nourishing your body with nutrients that restore vibrant life to your cells.

CHAPTER TWENTY

FORGIVENESS

More than twenty years ago, I created whimsical sculptures that caught the attention of an investor named John. John offered to become my business partner and market the sculptures as a toy line.

Before I knew it, we were romantically involved and he had become actively involved in my young daughter's life. As time went on, the reality of business pressures and personality differences set in. Emotionally unable to face him, I decided to end the relationship while he was out of town.

On his return, he expected me to greet him at the airport. Instead, he was forced to pay the hundred-mile cab fare home. Once he'd discovered I'd left him, he was enraged and determined to seek revenge. A few nights later, he barged into my house while I was sleeping and took my daughter!

The next few days are a complete blur. John would call intermittently to explain how he was saving my daughter from a terrible "me." He babbled almost incoherently.

After several nightmarish days, the FBI tracked him down. He was arrested and my daughter was returned to me.

I couldn't work. I couldn't think. The business we'd created together quickly fell apart. I was full of anger and bitterness—toward myself and toward John. It chipped away at my health, my mind, and my soul.

I turned to a priest at an Episcopal church—not that I was the least bit religious at the time. After listening to my story, he told me to list every unkind thing that I had done to John. I was confused and tried to make him understand that the problem wasn't me, it was John.

He replied, "I understand. Just make the list and return when you have finished."

I went home and started the list that grew and grew. I was astonished to see all of the terrible things I had done to hurt this man.

I returned to the church, weeping. After I finished reciting my list to the priest, he told me that I would be forgiven if I confessed my wrongdoings and asked God for forgiveness. Then, he told me to leave it all behind me.

When I walked out of the church, I felt peace. I felt clean, light, and joyful. The heavy burden had disappeared. My feelings of hatred and anger were replaced with love and remorse. I felt terrible about the way I'd treated John. Yes, his response to my action was very wrong, but I could now understand his reaction.

Forgiveness is the most important exercise in this book. No matter how well you eat and exercise, anger, hatred, and bitterness toward yourself or someone else can destroy your body and mind! Stress is the major cause of physical illness. Unforgiveness causes stress.

If you experience a life where people are hard on you, please look deep within yourself. Perhaps you are doing the same thing to others in thoughts, words, or deeds.

Glenda Green writes in *Love without End:*[1]

[E]xistence responds to the cause and effect of love rather than the cause and effect of action. Thus, a man may give to one and receive from another. He may selflessly give of his time to conserve nature and be rewarded by the teachings of life. He may visit the sick and be healed of his own self-pity. He may forgive one man and be forgiven by others.

I believe that the ability to forgive is the result of a deep gratitude for life. In order to forgive, we must rise above and let go.

FORGIVENESS EXERCISE

Step One

Do you harvest what you sow? This exercise is based on the works of Henry W. Wright, from his book *A More Excellent Way*, about the spiritual roots of disease.

Look over the following list and answer the questions:

1. Seeds of Unforgiveness: Do you experience an emotional charge when you think of a person who has hurt you?

2. Growth of Resentment: Do you find yourself talking or thinking about the list of the wrongs committed by a person toward you or someone you care about? Does it happen often? Has it increased in intensity?

3. Vine of Retaliation: Do you find yourself thinking about ways to get even with this person? Do you find yourself being passive-aggressive toward this person, acting sarcastically toward him/her, or talking about this person to others? Do you purposely do "little" things to get even? Do you enjoy knowing when this person experiences a bit of suffering in his/her life?

4. Thorns of Anger: Are your feelings toward this person charged with anger? Are you obsessed with your anger for this person? (People often find themselves pushing others away by telling the story of the wrong inflicted on them by another person.)

5. Weeds of Hatred: Can you tolerate the presence of this person without experiencing hatred or disgust? (This is different from choosing to avoid someone.) With hatred, even the thought of being around this person sets off a strong emotional charge.

6. Blight of Violence: This is when you want someone who has wronged you to feel emotional or physical pain.

7. Total Destruction: This is when you act out to destroy another person's life, reputation, property, or mental state. Total destruction of a relationship is often experienced during divorce.

Step Two

Looking at the inappropriate thoughts and behaviors you have toward someone else, regardless of what they have done to you, is a great tool for discovering what you're hiding in your heart. As God's children, we should always focus on the things we can control in our own lives—not focus on controlling the actions and behaviors of others.

- Make a list of the wrongdoings you've refused to forgive.

- Make a list of your wrongdoings inflicted upon each person that you have not forgiven.

- Allow yourself to feel the pain of the wrongdoings as you inflicted them.

- Read the list aloud, preferably to someone you trust.

- Ask God for help to forgive and release these feelings.

If the emotional charge is too overwhelming, I suggest you get spiritual or professional help.

CHAPTER TWENTY-ONE

NURTURING

Tell me what you eat and I will tell you what you are.
—Jean-Anthelme Brillat-Savarin

Eating was never meant to be a source of emotional nurturing. God meant for us to obtain comfort from satisfying relationships and meaningful work. In today's culture, we get wrapped up in the "material" things of life: wealth, power, achievement, duty, and so on. When disappointed, we seek comfort and escape from these "material" things. Food is an easy but disappointing way to feed the malnourished soul.

As you eat the Super Antioxidant Diet way, you should begin to unravel your relationship with food. You will also experience more mental clarity and heightened awareness.

Try the following exercise after you have been following this plan for about a month and see what you experience.

EXERCISE: FEEDING THE MALNOURISHED SOUL

Think back to your early childhood. Focus on the joyful memories, not the traumatic ones. What made life fascinating to you? What absorbed you so much that you completely lost track of time? Was it creating a talent show, drawing a picture, gazing up into the night sky, or listening to music? Was it building a fort, playing catch, collecting rocks, or sitting in a tree swing? There are clues in these memories. You may find activities you forgot you enjoyed. You may even recognize a forgotten calling.

Focus on recapturing the peace and joyful excitement of these activities. Mentally visualize those happy times.

Pondering these memories can help you recreate activities that are healthy and nurturing. Then, actively seek situations and opportunities that make you happy and laugh. Experiencing a positive environment will help diminish your emotional craving for food.

CHAPTER TWENTY-TWO

ATTITUDE

*The way you think, the way you behave, and the way you eat
can influence your life for thirty to fifty years.*
—Deepak Chopra

When we face stressful situations, our brain triggers powerful chemicals that prepare us for confrontation or escape. If we encounter stress often, this reaction takes on a sense of normalcy.

With a positive attitude, we can conquer the inclination to be stressed, tense, and upset. Change takes practice, however.

EXERCISE ONE:
ATTITUDE ANCHOR

• What is the most blissful moment you have ever experienced?

• Do you remember how you felt at that moment?

• Etch that moment and feeling into your brain. This is your Attitude Anchor.

During times of stress or tension, remember your Attitude Anchor, and practice focusing on it often.

EXERCISE TWO:
ATTITUDE LIVING

This exercise focuses on the attributes of others. Work it into everything you do, and you will find a sense of fulfillment.

• Look for positive attributes in every person you encounter.

• When you become bored or idle, make a mental list of the positive attributes of people you know.

- Take the time to listen to everyone you know and find ways to acknowledge their feelings. Perhaps someone is praising a grandchild's accomplishments or simply trying to choose a color to paint the kitchen. Make a mental note of whatever is important to that person at that moment, and reference it the next time you see him/her.

- Affirm the improvements or accomplishments of people you know no matter how insignificant they may seem.

- Make an effort to randomly help others in need.

CHAPTER TWENTY-THREE

SOCIAL PRESSURE

Even with the tools you have learned so far, you will face bad days and temptations to choose non-life-altering actions. I used to crave comfort food after a stressful day, and the desire for those quick fixes became overpowering at times. I would imagine the taste of my mother's roast beef and rich mashed potatoes, then rush to replicate that feeling with some type of food.

Many people use food to nurture those they love. They may not know any other way to show affection. Perhaps it's a potluck party, dinner at a friend's house, a family reunion, or a church social. We all have those people who insist we enjoy a huge piece of their special dish. How do you say no without that person feeling rejected?

You may have had a horrible day and your best friend insists you enjoy her freshly baked, gooey brownies with a dollop of Ben and Jerry's ice cream on top. The friend is very important to you. Do you want to reject her for offering comfort? What do you do? Run for the door as fast as you can? Get angry with her for tempting you?

Maybe it's the overweight grandmother who cooks all the time. Maybe she makes comments like: "You deserve a little treat because you've been working so hard lately." Or "I made this just for you, and now you won't try even a tiny piece?"

Stressful situations, social situations, food ritual habits . . . how do we break the chain? If in a social situation, simply acknowledge your appreciation, lovingly explain your need to make a healthy choice, and divert the discussion away from food. If alone, step back from the situation and acknowledge your power and purpose. Do your exercises, and remember that changing a behavior takes practice.

Read the following examples and the questions you should ask yourself when facing food temptation.

Example One

Question: What are you feeling?

Possible Response: Jittery and excited.

Question: What are the thoughts telling you?

Possible Response: I've been eating very healthfully and I feel great! Now I deserve a treat!

Question: Is that really the best choice you can make? Why do you want to reward yourself with saturated fat, sugar, stimulants, and processed flour—foods that you now know lead to sickness and death. What kind of reward is that?

Example Two

Question: What are you feeling?

Possible Response: Uncomfortable. If I say no, I'll hurt her feelings.

Question: Is it better to set a healthy example for you both or not take the chance of hurting feelings?

Example Three

Question: What are you feeling?

Possible Response: If I say no, I'll be the only one in the group not eating this food. I'm afraid I won't fit in if I don't eat like everyone else!

Question: Is your involvement with this group based on who you are as a human being or how you eat?

Example Four

Question: What are you feeling?

Possible Response: If I say no, I'm afraid I'll sound preachy. I'm the only one trying to get healthy. I don't want to seem better than everyone else.

Question: Do you have to make a huge deal by saying no? Just take small portions and pick at the food. Get involved in the conversation instead. Did you eat something healthy before you arrived so you wouldn't be tempted?

In today's society, food is often the centerpiece of social activities. We also know that people influence each other with their habits and lifestyles. If the foundation of a relationship in your life is to participate in an unhealthy behavior, you might need to reevaluate that relationship. Most people are unwilling to give up negative habits and they may hinder your growth (either consciously or unconsciously).

Until your new lifestyle becomes easier for you, it may be best to separate yourself from the people who might hinder you. At a later time, when you are stronger, you might be able to influence them by modeling a healthy lifestyle.

Becoming quiet and fully experiencing life opens the door for new relationships and activities. You might consider volunteering, learning an art or craft, taking a continuing education class, joining a walking group, or participating in neighborhood gardening. In this way, you can meet new people with whom you share healthy interests.

As you continue to gain strength and become healthier, remember to respect others. Make sure that you do not become critical of people who lack willpower or self-esteem. Make sure you do not judge people for being overweight like you once felt people judged you. After all, you can only control *your own* behavior.

APPENDIX I

JUST MOVE! BARE MINIMUM FITNESS

Physical fitness is not only one of the most important keys to a healty body,
it is the basis of dynamic and creative intellectual activity.
—John F. Kennedy

I have unpleasant memories associated with exercise. Although extremely coordinated on a horse, I dreaded school team sports and was always the last one chosen. In college, I was determined to overcome my shy awkwardness, so I took beginning jazz dance. My teacher felt sorry for me and suggested I drop out, but I stuck with it. She seemed horrified when I returned to take the course over again!

Throughout the years, I have continued to work on balance and coordination. It's gotten easier. I take courses that require learning steps and movements. Eating a high-nutrient diet and following a regular exercise routine also helps me focus, which in turn helps balance and coordination. Now that I've given up training horses, I try to walk at least four miles four times a week.

Many of us make excuses not to exercise: "I don't have the time or energy to do one more thing," "I have to take the kids to practice," "My joints hurt too much," "I'm eating better; that should count, right?" Sound familiar?

Like everything else in this book, we must make the commitment to learn new behaviors by making different choices. Make the commitment to exercise.

You may want to begin only with a comfortable walk three or four times per week. After six weeks and substantial weight loss, you may be ready to ease into a moderate exercise program. Do not expect to suddenly become an athlete. Impossible expectations and attempting too many sudden changes are recipes for failure.

Whatever exercise you choose, consult your doctor if you have not exercised in several years and are more than thirty pounds overweight. The benefits of exercise include:

• General feeling of health and well-being

• Greater physical work capacity

• Relief from tension

• Less fatigue

• Improved neuromuscular skill and physical performance

• Improved posture and appearance

• Stimulation of mental activity

• Controlled body weight

• Prevention, delay, or a greater ability to withstand and recover from cardiovascular disease and other diseases

• Prevention of pain in the lower back

• Delayed aging process

• Better digestion and bowel movements

• Improved functioning of the internal organs

Dr. Couey, a cellular physiologist and world-renowned nutrition and fitness expert, designed Bare Minimum Fitness to help you ease into an exercise program.

BARE MINIMUM FITNESS, by Dr. Richard B. Couey

GUIDELINES

Regular cardiovascular exercise and weight training promote physical, mental, psychological, and social fitness. They can be a great release from tension. They promote self-confidence and positive social interaction.

Probably the worst thing you can do to begin your cardiovascular program is grab your old tennis shoes, head for the nearest track, and run at top speed. You must prepare yourself physically before you rush into any cardiovascular exercise. Otherwise, someone may have to rush you to the hospital!

I recommend you get a medical exam prior to beginning an exercise program, especially if you are older than thirty-five.

The examination should consist of standard and stress electrocardiograms (ECGs); resting and exercise blood pressure measurements; fasting blood sugar (glucose), cholesterol, triglyceride, and high-density lipoprotein determinations; and evaluation of any orthopedic problem.

Here are some simple guidelines that will help protect you from harm and injury:

Warm up before exercising. Prepare your body with a proper warm-up prior to exercising. The warm-up is a precaution against unnecessary injuries and muscle soreness. It also stimulates the heart and lungs moderately and progressively, as well as increases the blood flow and the blood and muscle temperatures gradually. It prepares you mentally for taking action, too.

A five-minute warm-up routine is recommended to stretch the arms, legs, and back. After stretching, start warming up by walking at your regular pace. Walk flat-footed as much as possible during the warm-up. This gives the tendons and ligaments in the feet and ankles a chance to stretch gradually, helping to avoid possible irritation from sudden stress.

The time required for warm-up varies with each individual. Sweat indicates that the core temperature has increased and more intense conditioning can be done. Keep in mind that cold weather requires longer warm-up times.

Cool down after exercising. Cooling down after completing the cardiovascular activity is as important to the body as the warm-up. During the exercise, the large muscles of the legs provide a boost to the circulating blood and help return it to the heart and lungs where the change of oxygen and carbon dioxide takes place. As the muscles relax after exertion, blood fills the veins. It is not allowed to flow backward because of the valves in the veins. During exercise, the squeezing action of the leg muscles provides about half of the pumping action, while the heart provides the other half. A slower paced walk allows the muscle pump to continue until the total volume of blood is decreased to the point the heart can handle it without help from the muscles.

Always reduce your exercise pace very slowly, never abruptly. Do not stop instantly or sit down after vigorous exercise. The blood will pool in your legs and result in lack of blood to the brain.

Exercise within your tolerance range. Do not push yourself to the extent of becoming overly tired. This is not only dangerous to your health, but also defeats the purpose of exercise. If your body does not feel strong when you first awake, you may be overtraining.

Progress slowly. Moving too quickly invites trouble such as muscle and joint injuries. Gradually work up to your exercise goals.

Get adequate rest and nutrition. No matter how hard or long you train, you will not achieve optimal results without proper nutrition and rest.

Exercise regularly. Consistency and regularity are necessary for optimal benefits. Spasmodic exercise can be dangerous. For every one week you skip exercise, it takes nearly two weeks to return to your previous fitness level. Just as we have to replenish our nutrition daily, we have to exercise regularly to reap the benefits of exercise.

Wear the proper shoes. A worn-out, cheaply made, or poorly fitting pair of shoes can cause foot, leg, and hip injuries. Proper shoes eliminate many of the hazards associated with walking such as blisters and stress to the feet, legs, and hips. Canvas tennis shoes are not good for walking because they are too heavy and provide poor support for the ligaments and bones. I recommend you purchase the best shoes you can possibly afford. Anyone unsure about what shoes to purchase would be wise to consult with someone who exercises regularly.

Exercise cautiously in hot weather. Never exercise vigorously when the combined temperature and humidity reach 165 or above (for example, 85 degrees Fahrenheit and 80 percent humidity). Exercising in this type of heat increases the susceptibility to heat stroke. The best method of cooling your body during exercise is through evaporation. If the humidity is above 80 percent, the evaporative process in the body will not function properly, because a humid atmosphere cannot accept more moisture—including the moisture coming from the body. Body temperature will quickly rise, instead.

If you live in a hot and humid climate, you may need to exercise early in the morning or late at night. Wear clothes that allow your body to cool itself by evaporation. Never wear a sweat suit or rubberized suit. Do not try to lose weight by sweating. This is dangerous. You will also gain the weight back when you drink fluids.

Dress appropriately in cold conditions. Most people overdress when they exercise in cold temperatures. Dress to feel comfortably warm during the exercise period without profusely sweating. Usually, one or two layers of light clothing, a knit cap covering the head and ears, and knit gloves are sufficient. In very cold weather, a ski mask can be worn to protect the face and warm the air as it goes into the lungs. Always walk with the wind in the latter stage of your exercise. The chill factor is increased when you walk briskly into the wind. If you walk against the wind after sweating has increased, the chilling effects of the wind will be magnified.

This fitness plan is designed like an à la carte menu. Choose whatever types of cardiovascular exercises you prefer, and exercise four times a week. Include an easy weight-resistance exercise three times a week, which can even be done at the same time.

Menu Choices for Cardiovascular Health

Walking

If you have been inactive for four weeks or longer, start with a walking program to slowly develop your leg muscles, ligaments, and tendons. For older adults or those with a low level of cardiovascular fitness, walking provides enough physical stress to increase cardiovascular fitness. If you are in poor physical condition because of prior inactivity or obesity, follow these suggestions:

• Map out a one-mile scenic route by your car's odometer. You don't have to walk a full mile in the beginning, just walk at a normal, easy, steady pace. Swing your arms rhythmically, take in a deep breath on every fifth breath and release the air as much as possible. Make sure to land on your heel first at foot strike.

• Talk to someone while walking. If you can't carry on a short conversation, you may be walking too fast for your present fitness level. If you are not slightly winded while talking, then you should increase your pace.

• Increase your speed to a fifteen-minute mile after several weeks of walking. If you cannot maintain a brisk pace, periodically slow up for several seconds, then return to your more intense pace.

Bicycling

To achieve a training effect with a bicycle, map out a safe route with your odometer. To receive the necessary heart benefits, try cycling about ten to twelve miles per hour. Also, warm up by cycling slowly for three minutes before attempting the specified time. Cool down by cycling slowly for three minutes at the conclusion of exercise.

Stationary Cycling

For those unable to walk or swim because of orthopedic problems, the stationary exercise bike provides a good stimulus for the cardiovascular system.

The bicycle seat should be high enough so that the extended leg in the down position is almost straight. Warm up by cycling for three minutes at zero resistance, and cool down at the conclusion of the exercise in the same way.

MENU CHOICES FOR HEALTHY WEIGHT TRAINING

Strong muscles are synonymous with healthy bones. Following the Super Antioxidant Diet will help you achieve your ideal slender weight, but simply following the most nutrient-dense diet is not enough to protect most women from osteoporosis. Being slender usually makes a person more prone to osteoporosis, because lighter bodies create less weight resistance for the muscles.

A basic weight-training program should strengthen all major muscle groups in a balanced manner. It is unhealthy to strengthen one part of the body without strengthening other parts equally. Muscle imbalances can cause postural deviations and joint injuries. You must learn the proper lifting and breathing techniques before attempting a weight-lifting program.

Fancy equipment is not needed to start a good weight-training program, although using special weight-training machines found in private health clubs makes weight training very convenient! You can start gently by using an exercise band or lifting food cans. Another alternative is a weight vest, but even a weight vest can be dangerous if worn improperly or overloaded with weights.

Weight Training Do's and Don'ts

If you choose to participate in a weight-resistance program at a health club or use free weights at home, follow these important guidelines:

• Be prepared. Use rubber-soled shoes to avoid slipping and wear cotton clothing to absorb perspiration.

• Warm up. A whole body warm-up should always precede a regular weight workout. Walk briskly or perform light calisthenics until a light sweat appears.

• Breathe. Never hold your breath when exerting. Holding the breath causes drastic elevation in chest and abdominal pressure. Breathe!

• Start with a very light load. During the first week of training, use light weights to familiarize yourself with the movement and correct form for each exercise. This also prepares the muscles for a gradual increase in resistance. An experienced trainer can show you how to control the correct weight with a complete range of motion and proper form.

• Use the correct form. Correct form is essential for developing the body symmetrically and protecting the body from injury. Do not lift more than you can handle, even with good form. The amount lifted is not important, but rather how well each exercise is performed. Always keep your head up and back straight when lifting weights. Severe damage can occur to the discs in the spinal column when lifting with the back bent.

• Achieve the full range of motion. Failure to perform each exercise movement with the complete range of motion will result in partial development of the primary muscles and a corresponding loss of flexibility in the opposing muscles. This will cause a muscle-bound appearance.

• Lift weights regularly and proportionately. Perform weight-resistance exercises three times per week between cardiovascular workouts. You can develop alternating exercise routines of upper and lower body. A weight-training session should last thirty minutes,

although you may want to lengthen it to gain strength, endurance, and experience.

• Slowly increase number of repetitions for each weight-bearing exercise.

• Month one: One set of 10 reps

• Month two: Two sets of 10 reps

• Month three: Three sets of 10 reps

FLEXIBILITY

Flexibility promotes health. With age, our bodies tend to become more restricted in bending, stretching, and reaching up high. If we were to return to the school playground and attempt to go through the motions of the past, most of us would be unable to perform them.

Flexibility differs from one person to the next because of joint and bone structure, muscle amount, and the amount of fatty tissue around joints. A flexibility program, no matter how good, cannot change basic joint structure. It can, however, stretch the muscles, ligaments, and connective tissue that surround a joint.

Flexibility is an important aspect of physical fitness, and the lack of it can create many health disorders. If you can't touch your toes with your legs straight, you greatly increase your chances of developing lower back pain. A stiff spinal column can also cause postural problems. Lack of flexibility can also be responsible for muscle injury, compression of nerves, severe headaches, and even some forms of arthritis.

What Type of Stretching Is Best?

Stretching feels good and is great for the body! Avoid fast, jerky, bouncy movements because they cause the muscles you are attempting to stretch to contract at the same time. This not only reduces the effectiveness of stretching, but also increases the risks of injury and muscle soreness.

Slow, static stretching seems to cause far less muscle soreness. In fact, a slow, gradual static stretch can relieve muscle soreness. Stretch receptors located in the muscles and joints are stimulated by specific kinds of stretching movements. They protect the muscles and joints from overstretching and injuring themselves. When a slow, sustained stretch is used, the stretch receptors cause the muscle to relax and lengthen, and thus aid in obtaining increased flexibility.

APPENDIX II

THE SUPER ANTIOXIDANT DIET AND YOUR DOG

Chippy, my fifteen-year-old dachshund, was once obese and lethargic. I put him on a modified Super Antioxidant Diet about a year and a half ago.

I first introduced fruits and vegetables cooked in a stew while I slowly cut back on commercial dog food. He was a little finicky at first, but quickly developed a ravenous appetite for healthy plant foods. On his new diet plan, he not only lost weight but also regained his youthful vigor.

One week, I went out of town and left Chippy with my parents, who do not have a yard. It was inconvenient for them to take him out regularly. Increased plant food intake had caused an increase in his bowel movements. After a few indoor accidents, they decided to give him commercial dog food. As a result, he became very ill and stopped eating.

After I returned, I immediately took him to the vet where I learned that poor kidney function had caused him to become severely dehydrated. Nonetheless, the doctor said his other organs were unusually healthy for a dog his age.

The vet suggested an expensive rehydration treatment, but it failed. At that point, he didn't believe Chippy could be saved and suggested euthanasia. I refused to give up and took Chippy home. My parents were devastated and suggested I get another opinion.

Dad and I took Chippy to another vet who saw just how healthy his organs were, in spite of his kidney problems. She suggested a vegan diet with lots of vegetables and fruits but no animal protein because it might tax his kidneys. She also commented that Chippy had early-stage cataracts. We were to return in six weeks. I left with little hope.

I prepared a special super antioxidant mixture and added Pedialyte (an electrolyte solution formulated for children). I froze the mixture in individual daily servings. To ensure he was getting all the nutrients he needed, I supplemented the homemade mixture with a small portion of high-quality commercial dog food.

At first, Chippy didn't have much appetite, but in a couple of days, his appetite increased and the sparkle in his eyes returned.

After six weeks, he was completely renewed. His kidney functions were vastly imrpoved and he had no signs of cataracts. Chippy, who had almost been euthanized, had returned to my healthy and happy "best friend." I often wonder how he would be if I had fed him this healthy diet his whole life. Would other dogs' life spans be longer if fed this diet? I decided to research the most popular pet foods and their ingredients.

Immediately, I discovered that most pet foods contain chemical preservatives and by-products that are unfit for human consumption. Sadly, there is no government agency to watch over the pet food industry. So our precious pets depend on us to feed them the healthiest diet.

The fact is: I unknowingly fed Chippy chemical preservatives, animal by-products, and unhealthy fillers by giving him commercial dog food. So become educated and make your own decision!

The following list of unhealthy ingredients often found in dog foods is also available on the Flint River Ranch pet food website (www.frrinc.com):

1. Corn Products: Corn Meal, Corn Gluten Meal, Corn Oil: Corn is indigestible to dogs, due to their short intestines.

2. Chicken By-Products: Ingredients listed as animal by-products are not required to include actual meat. Chicken by-products may include intestines, chicken heads, feathers, bone, beaks, and feet.

3. Dried Egg Products: Ingredients listed as product may include an unspecified part of the product. Egg product may include eggshells, and may also not include any egg whites.

4. Natural Chicken Flavor: Any flavor added reflects the lack of flavor in the main food ingredients.

5. Soybean Meal: Soybean meal is used as a filler product and has little or no nutritional value.

6. BHA/BHT: These ingredients are chemical preservatives that have been banned for human use in many countries. Their use in pet foods is still allowed in the United States.

Because Chippy and other dogs have experienced amazing results on an antioxidant diet, I wanted to give you the opportunity to feed your dog the recipe that helped Chippy.

You can also keep up with all of my antioxidant information by visiting www.vibrantcuisine.com. Please write or email me about how the Super Antioxidant Diet helps you, your loved ones, and even your dog. Enjoy!

SUPER ANTIOXIDANT DOG FOOD
Yield: Approximately 14 pounds

1 cup regular rolled oats
1 cup brown rice
1 pound lentils
2 pounds frozen chopped collard greens
1 pound frozen chopped broccoli
1 pound frozen peas and carrots
1 pound frozen okra
1 pound green beans
12 to 16 cups water
1 pound frozen blueberries
½ pound mixed berries
1 cup nutritional yeast
½ cup freshly ground flaxseed
2 pounds raw free-range chicken (skinned), or wild game, or range-fed beef or buffalo

In a 2-gallon kettle, cover and simmer all ingredients except berries, yeast, flaxseed, and raw meat for 1 hour. Stir occasionally and add more water if necessary to keep from scorching. Remove from heat and cool. Mix in berries, yeast, and flax. Chill in refrigerator or freeze in one pound servings.

Serve with some raw meat. Older dogs require less meat because nitrogen can tax their kidneys.

Mix in grated or finely chopped fresh fruit and raw vegetables to add antioxidants with live enzymes. This aids digestion.

Add a small amount of a high-quality fortified dog food such as Flint River Ranch to ensure that your dog gets vitamins and minerals.

My 19-pound dachshund needs about 2 cups per day plus ¼ cup high-quality dried dog food and 2 tablespoons raw ground buffalo meat.

Warning: Do not give your dog grapes, raisins, onion, garlic, chocolate, caffeine, or alcohol.

ENDNOTES

Chapter 1

1. Quoted in Quillen, Patrick. *Beating Cancer with Nutrition.* Tulsa, OK: Nutrition Times Press, 1998, p 84.
2. Jacob RA, Burri BJ. "Oxidative damage and defense." *Am J Clin Nutr* 1996; 63(6):985S–990S.
3. Waladkhani AR, Clemens MR. "Effect of dietary phytochemicals on cancer development." In RR Watson (ed). *Vegetables, Fruits, and Herbs in Health Promotion.* Boca Raton, FL: CRC Press, 2001, pp 147–176.
4. O'Neill KL, et al. "Fruits and vegetables and the prevention of oxidative DNA damage." In RR Watson (ed). *Vegetables, Fruits, and Herbs in Health Promotion.* Boca Raton, FL: CRC Press, 2001, pp 135–146.
5. Ingram DK, et al. "Development of calorie restriction mimetics as a prolongevity strategy." *Ann NY Acad Sci.* 2004;1019: 412–423.
6. Heilbronn LK, et al. "Effect of 6-month calorie restriction on biomarkers of longevity, metabolic adaptation, and oxidative stress in overweight individuals: A randomized controlled trial." *JAMA* 2006;295(13):1539–1548.
7. Fontana L, et al. "Long-term calorie restriction is highly effective in reducing the risk for atherosclerosis in humans." *Proc Natl Acad Sci USA.* 2004;101(17): 6659–6663.
8. Waladkhani AR, Clemens MR. "Effect of dietary phytochemicals on cancer development." In RR Watson (ed). *Vegetables, Fruits, and Herbs in Health Promotion.* Boca Raton, FL: CRC Press, 2001, pp 147–176.
9. O'Neill KL, et al. "Fruits and vegetables and the prevention of oxidative DNA damage." In RR Watson (ed). *Vegetables, Fruits, and Herbs in Health Promotion.* Boca Raton, FL: CRC Press, 2001, pp 135–146.

Chapter 2

1. Heald Claire. "Going Ape." *BBC News Magazine,* January 1, 2007, news.bbc.co.uk/2/hi/uk_news/magazine/6248975.stm.
2. Peary W, Peavy W. "Natural toxins in sprouted seeds: Separating myth from reality." *Vegetarian J* 1995;14(4):17–20.
3. Yang A, et al. "Warmed-over flavor and lipid stability of beef: Effects of prior nutrition." *J Food Sci* 2002;67(9): 3309–3313.
4. Chilton, Floyd H. *Inflammation Nation.* New York: Fireside, 2005, pp 114–116.
5. Miles EA, Calder PC. "Modulation of immune function by dietary fatty acids." *Proc Nutr Soc* 1998;63(2):341–349.
6. Shankar A, et al. "Association between circulating white blood cell count and cancer mortality: A population-based cohort study." *Arch Intern Med* 2006; 166:188–194.
7. Chilton, Floyd H. *Inflammation Nation.* New York: Fireside, 2005, p 86.
8. Weaver CM, Plawecki KL. "Dietary calcium: Adequacy of a vegetarian diet." *Am J Clin Nutr* 1994;59(5 Suppl):1238S–1241S.
9. Kelemen LE, et al. "Vegetables, fruit, and antioxidant-related nutrients and risk of

non-Hodgkin lymphoma: A National Cancer Institute–Surveillance, Epidemiology, and End Results population-based case-control study." *Am J Clin Nutr* 2006;83(6):1401–1410.

10. Zhang Y, et al. "A major inducer of anti-carcinogenic protective enzymes from broccoli: Isolation and elucidation of structure." *Proc Natl Acad Sci USA* 1992;89(6):2399–2403.

11. Conaway CC, et al. "Disposition of glucosinolates and sulforaphane in humans after ingestion of steamed and fresh broccoli. *Nutr Cancer* 2000;38(2):168–178.

12. Nestle M. "Broccoli sprouts as inducers of carcinogen-detoxifying enzyme systems: Clinical, dietary, and policy implications." *Proc Natl Acad Sci USA* 1997;94(21):11149–11151.

13. McIntosh M. "A diet containing food rich in soluble and insoluble fiber improves glycemic control and reduces hyperlipidemia among patients with type 2 diabetes mellitus." *Nutr Rev* 2001;59(2):52–55.

14. Jenkins DJ, et al. "Exceptionally low blood glucose response to dried beans: Comparison with other carbohydrate foods." *Br Med J* 1980;281(6240):578–580.

15. Joseph JA, et al. "Reversals of age-related declines in neuronal signal transduction, cognitive, and motor behavioral deficits with blueberry, spinach, or strawberry dietary supplementation." *J Neurosci* 1999;19(18):8114–8121.

16. Aviram M, et al. "Pomegranate juice flavonoids inhibit low-density lipoprotein oxidation and cardiovascular diseases: Studies in atherosclerotic mice and in humans." *Drugs Exp Clin Res* 2002;28(2–3):49–62.

17. de Nigris F, et al. "Beneficial effects of pomegranate juice on oxidation-sensitive genes and endothelial nitric oxide synthase activity at sites of perturbed sheer stress." *Proc Natl Acad Sci USA* 2005;102(13):4896–4901.

18. Lovgren S. "US Racking Up Huge 'Sleep Debt.'" *National Geographic News* 2005(Feb 24). news.nationalgeographic.com/news/2005/02/0224_sleep.html.

Chapter 3

1. Couey R. *Nutrition for God's Temple.* Dyfed, Wales: The Edwin Mellen Press, Ltd. Lampeter, 1993.

2. Campbell TC. *The China Study.* Dallas, Texas: First Bella Books, 2004.

3. Protein combining, from Wikipedia, the free encyclopedia: Protein combining (also *protein complementing*) is the theory, now largely discredited, that vegetarians must eat foods such as beans and rice together, or at least on the same day, so the different amino acids in the foods combine to form a "complete" protein, containing all eight essential amino acids necessary for human growth and maintenance. In fact, all essential amino acids are present in common individual plant foods, including beans, rice, potatoes, and corn.

4. Lappe FM. *Diet for a Small Planet*, 10th anniversary edition. New York: Ballantine Books, 1982.

5. Lipton BH. *The Biology of Belief.* Santa Rosa, CA: Mountain of Love/Elite Books, 2005, p 171.

6. Couey R. *Nutrition for God's Temple.* Dyfed, Wales: The Edwin Mellen Press, Ltd. Lampeter, 1993, p 242.

7. Lisle DJ, Goldhamer A. *The Pleasure Trap.* Summertown, TN: Healthy Living Publications, 2003, p 9.

Chapter 5

1. "Repaying Your Sleep Debt." *Harvard Women's Health Watch* newsletter, July 2007.
2. "Repaying Your Sleep Debt." *Harvard Women's Health Watch* newsletter, July 2007.
3. Dzugan SA. "Natural strategies for managing insomnia." *Life Extension* 2006(Dec):77.
4. Howenstine, James, MD. January 15, 2004; NewsWithViews.com.
5. Holick MF. "Vitamin D and health in the 21st century: Bone and beyond." *Am J Clin Nutr* 2004;80(6):1678S–1688S.
6. Spahr A, et al. "Periodontal infections and coronary heart disease role of periodontal bacteria and importance of total pathogen burden in the Coronary Event and Periodontal Disease (CORODONT) Study." *Arch Intern Med* 2006;166(5): 554–559.

Chapter 6

1. Couey R. *Nutrition for God's Temple.* Dyfed, Wales: The Edwin Mellen Press, Ltd. Lampeter, 1993, p 146.
2. Khan N, et al. "Pomegranate fruit extract inhibits prosurvival pathways in human A549 lung carcinoma cells and tumor growth in athymic nude mice." *Carcinogenesis* 2007;28(1):163–173.
3. Pantuck AJ, et al. "Phase II study of pomegranate juice for men with rising prostate-specific antigen following surgery or radiation for prostate cancer." *Clin Cancer Res* 2006;12(13):4018–4026.

4. Jeune MA, et al. "Anticancer activities of pomegranate extracts and genistein in human breast cancer cells." *Angiogenesis* 2003;6(2):121–128.

Chapter 7

1. Joossens JV, et al. "Dietary salt, nitrate and stomach cancer mortality in 24 countries: European Cancer Prevention (ECP) and the INTERSALT Cooperative Research Group." *Int J Epidemiol* 1996;25(3):494–504.
2. Itoh R, Suyama Y. "Sodium excretion in relation to calcium and hydroxproline excretion in a healthy Japanese population." *Am J Clin Nutr* 1996;63(5): 735–740.
3. Bragg Liquid Amino Acids contains amino acid excitotoxins, which are neurotransmitters that can affect how we feel. Excitotoxins are found naturally in the brain. If excitotoxins are consumed in large quantities, they can disrupt brain function. The small amounts I recommend in the recipes should not affect you adversely. If you are extremely sensitive to MSG, you might want to avoid liquid aminos. MSG is the excitotoxin glutamate.
4. Phukan RK, et al. "Role of dietary habits in the development of esophageal cancer in Assam, the north-eastern region of India." *Nutr Cancer* 2001;39(2):204–209.
5. National Foundation for Cancer Research, NFCR Cancer Information Center; http://www2.nfcr.org/site/Page Server? pagename=cancers_esophageal.

Chapter 12

1. O'Keefe SJ, et al. "Why do African Americans get more colon cancer than

Native Africans?" *J Nutr* 2007;137(1 Suppl):175S–182S.

2. Hughes MC, et al. "Food intake and risk of squamous cell carcinoma of the skin in a community: The Nambour skin cancer cohort study." *Int J Cancer* 2006; 119(8):1953–1960.

3. Albert CM, et al. "Fish consumption and risk of sudden cardiac death." *JAMA* 1998;279(1):23–28.

4. He K, et al. "Fish consumption and risk of stroke in men." *JAMA* 2002;288(4): 3130–3136.

5. Campbell TC, et al. *Diet, Life-Style and Mortality in China: A Study of the Characteristics of 65 Chinese Countries.* Ithaca, NY: Oxford University Press, 1990.

6. Esselstyn CB, et al. "A strategy to arrest and reverse coronary artery disease: A 5-year longitudinal study of a single physician's practice." *J Fam Pract* 1995;41(6): 560–568.

7. Barnes PJ, et al. "Induction of cyclo-oxygenase-2 by cytokines in human cultured airway smooth muscle cells: Novel inflammatory role of this cell type." *Br J Pharmacol* 1997;120(5):910–916.

8. Yang A, et al. "Warmed-over flavor and lipid stability of beef: Effects of prior nutrition." *J Food Sci* 2002;67(9): 3309–3313.

9. Chilton, Floyd H. *Inflammation Nation.* New York: Fireside, 2005.

10. Das UN. "Cox-2 inhibitors and metabolism of essential fatty acids." *Med Sci Monit* 2005;11(7):RA233–237.

11. Li D, et al. "Contribution of meat fat to dietary arachidonic acid." *Lipids* 1998; 33(4):437–440.

Chapter 15

1. Lipton, Bruce H. *The Biology of Belief.* Santa Rosa, CA: Mountain of Love/Elite Books, 2005.

Chapter 17

1. Farhi, Donna. *The Breathing Book.* New York: Henry Holt, 1996.

2. Gluck ME, Geliebter A, Lorence M. "Cortisol stress response is positively correlated with central obesity in obese women with binge eating disorder (BED) before and after cognitive-behavioral treatment." *Ann NY Acad Sci* 2004; 1032:202–207.

3. Epel ES, et al. "Stress and body shape: Stress-induced cortisol secretion is consistently greater among women with central fat." *Psychosom Med* 2000;62(5):623–632.

4. Perricone, Nicholas. *Dr. Perricone's 7 Secrets to Beauty, Health, and Longevity: The Miracle of Cellular Rejuvenation.* New York: Ballantine Books, 2006.

Chapter 18

1. Gladwell, Malcolm. *Blink.* New York: Little, Brown, 2005.

Chapter 20

1. Green, Glenda. *Love without End.* Sedona, AZ: Spirits, 2002.

RESOURCES

STAY INFORMED

It is so important to keep up with exciting cutting-edge nutritional information. New studies are revealing fascinating findings every day. Learning these facts plays a big role in staying motivated during your transition. The following are some excellent resources to help you stay informed and motivated.

Academy for Coaching Excellence
www.academyforcoachingexcellence.com

Brassica Protection Products LLC
www.brassica.com

Caldwell B. Esselstyn Jr, MD
www.heartattackproof.com

Joel Fuhrman, MD
www.drfuhrman.com

Hallelujah Acres
www.hacres.com

Life Extension Foundation
www.lef.org

Gary Null
www.garynull.com

Nutrientrich
www.nutrientrich.com

Nutrition Advocate
www.nutritionadvocate.com
Dr. T. Colin Campbell's website champions nutrition and health.

John Robbins Healthy at 100
www.healthyat100.org

Vegsource.com
www.vegsource.com

RECOMMENDED BOOKS
(These books can be found in some libraries, most bookstores, and online.)

During your transition to a healthier lifestyle—until you get over the hump—I recommend that you immerse yourself in solid scientific evidence by reading what the pioneers and experts have to say. Submerging yourself in this subject matter will motivate you to stay on track. Repetition of the facts from a variety of angles will greatly assist you in internalizing this new way of life. It is helpful for your learning and transformation to share this new and exciting information. By doing this you help yourself and others.

Prescription for Dietary Wellness
Phyllis A. Balch, CNC

The China Study
T. Colin Campbell, PhD
(www.nutritionadvocate.com)

Prevent and Reverse Heart Disease
Caldwell Esselstyn Jr., MD
(www.heartattackproof.com)

The Breathing Book
Donna Farhi
(www.donnafarhi.co.nz)

Disease-Proof Your Child
Joel Fuhrman, MD
(www.drfuhrman.com)

Eat to Live
Joel Fuhrman, MD
(www.drfuhrman.com)

Fasting and Eating for Health
Joel Fuhrman, MD
(www.drfuhrman.com)

Blink
Malcolm Gladwell
(http://leighbureau.com/speaker.asp?id=77)

The Biology of Belief
Bruce H. Lipton, PhD
(www.brucelipton.com)

The Pleasure Trap
Douglas J. Lisle, PhD, and Alan Goldhamer, DC
(www.pleasuretrap.com)

The DNA of Healing
Margaret Ruby
(www.possibilitiesdna.com)

ABOUT THE AUTHORS

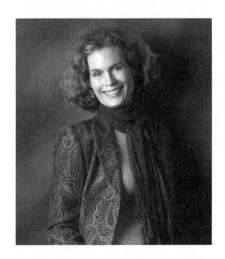

Robin Jeep first encountered exotic cooking as a child watching her mother cook. After moving to Europe to model and train as a steeplechase jockey, she discovered that a low-calorie, nutrient-rich diet would keep her thin, yet strong. During that time, she married a European prince and was given an opportunity to learn from great chefs around the world. She decided to use her knowledge to create mouth-watering cuisine that was both healthy and delicious.

Robin trained at the Culinary Institute of America at Greystone in Napa Valley, California. She apprenticed with Mike Maples of *Die Pupille* in Munich, Jeffrey Michaels of the *Royal Orleans* in New Orleans, and Executive Chef Piero of the famous *Toscana* in Los Angeles. She also served as director of marketing for Whole Foods in Dallas, where she transitioned it from a health food store to a more upscale, European-style market.

Later, while living in Los Angeles, Robin's creative flair with healthy food brought her to the attention of the founder of Private Chefs International (PCI), Christian Paier. PCI is a company that provides private chefs for top government officials, royalty, famous actors, and music stars. Robin worked as a private chef to many high-profile celebrities, including Jeff Lynne of the Electric Light Orchestra. She has also prepared healthy cuisine for celebrities such as Paul McCartney, Wendie Malick, Peter Max, Mikhail Baryshnikov, and Seal.

In 2002, Robin was the victim of a serious accident while horseback riding. The horse she was riding fell on top of her, fracturing fourteen pelvic bones, both of her hips, and her sacrum, and causing internal hemorrhaging. Her doctors had little hope for her, but she amazed them by being released from the hospital in record time. The doctors attributed Robin's miraculous and rapid recovery to her healthy lifestyle and nutrient-rich diet.

Robin considers the accident to be the biggest blessing of her life—a spiritual wakeup call—which gave her the chance to share a message of health and healing with others.

As founder of Vibrant Cuisine (a division of The Super Antioxidant Diet, LLC) Robin fuses health with international cuisines using antioxidant-rich ingredients. Through her lectures, workshops, and private consulting, she provides a holistic approach to nutritional education, personal growth, culinary instruction, physical fitness, and healthy social interaction. In addition, she and coauthor Richard Couey, PhD, have written a holistic curriculum for fitness centers and health clubs.

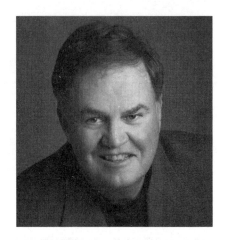

Dr. Richard Bryant Couey, PhD, has published more than twenty books on nutrition, fitness, wellness, spirituality, and golf. His most recent books are *Living Longer: The Magic of Enzymes and Nutrition*, which is a reference guide to the essentials of proper nutrition, and *The Happy Cell*, which explores how mind, body, and spirit can change body chemistry.

As a Professor at Baylor University for thirty-seven years, Couey specialized in exercise physiology, sports medicine, and nutrition. Prior to receiving his doctorate from Texas A&M University, Couey was a professional baseball player for the Chicago Cubs, worked as an exercise physiology consultant to the U.S. Olympic Team, and served as a member of the President's Commission on Physical Fitness and Sports. He has designed nutrition, fitness, and weight-loss programs for numerous wellness centers, police and fire departments, churches, and other groups such as the Texas Rangers Baseball Organization.

Couey is known nationally and internationally as a consultant and speaker on nutritional science and physical fitness issues.

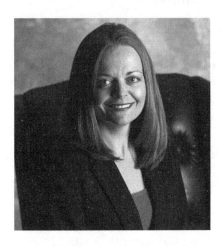

Sherie Ellington, the daughter of medical missionaries, spent her childhood in Nigeria, where she first witnessed the effects of poor nutrition. She combined her interests in health and nutrition with a career in communications and marketing, which she has done for more than twenty years. She has also freelanced as a weekly newspaper columnist and website designer, and has written numerous health-related articles. In her current position in economic development marketing near Dallas, Texas, she continues to be an advocate for healthy living. Her balanced lifestyle includes a positive attitude, nutritious diet, and regular exercise.

Sherie earned her AA in Commercial Art & Advertising from Texas State Technical College, graduated summa cum laude with a BA from the University of Texas at Arlington, and earned her MA from San Francisco State University.

Hampton Roads Publishing Company

. . . for the evolving human spirit

Hampton Roads Publishing Company
publishes books on a variety of subjects,
including spirituality, health, and other related topics.

For a copy of our latest trade catalog,
call toll-free, 800-766-8009,
or send your name and address to:

Hampton Roads Publishing Company, Inc.
1125 Stoney Ridge Road
Charlottesville, VA 22902
E-mail: hrpc@hrpub.com
Internet: www.hrpub.com